THE ENLIGHTENED GUIDE TO METHADONE MAINTENANCE TREATMENT

A Handbook for Navigating Opiate Addiction through Methadone Maintenance Treatment for Providers, Patients and their Families

KAY JOHN BORZSONY

ISBN: 9781654919313 (Paperback)

DEDICATION

This book is dedicated to all those opioid addicts who came before, and were forced to suffer unimaginable cruelty at the hands of greater society during a time when methadone treatment didn't yet exist. This book is also personally dedicated to those friends and family whose "time" came before me. They will forever be in my heart: Laszlo Borzsony, Eugene Borzsony, M.D., Randall Chuck, Jr., Todd Christian Fiore, and Judith Genette. May they all rest in peace and eternal justice.

ACKNOWLEDGEMENTS

I'd like to thank my wife, Maria, and my mother, Maren Swier-Bielenberg, for their unfailing support throughout the trying years of this project. I would be disingenuous were I not to acknowledge the disturbing *total and utter lack of interest* that this project created with whomever happened to be in my immediate radius, with the exception of fellow MMT patients. Considering that lives are at stake, it has repeatedly amazed me at how quick the majority of citizens are to dehumanize and devalue *anyone* with a substance abuse disorder, let alone opioid addiction.

TABLE OF CONTENTS

"It is the greatest achievement of a writer to irritate people."
Hamed Abdel-Samad

FOREWORD

The dawn of a new era is upon us, and that is the era of medication assisted treatment (MAT) for opioid addiction as a first-line treatment. Ever since the first methadone clinics opened in the early 1970s in the U.S., nothing in medicine has been the subject of more stigma, controversy, misinformation, and downright mythology than methadone maintenance treatment (MMT.) The stigma against MMT is staggering and well-known, and it is the primary intent of this text to eliminate all of the false myths and fears surrounding MMT by providing accurate, if not always politically correct information in an easy to understand format.

Before continuing, the American Society of Addiction Medicine (ASAM) lists three medications under the medication assisted treatment (MAT) rubric: methadone, buprenorphine, and naltrexone. The first two medications can, in our opinion, correctly be designated as medication assisted treatment whereas the third medication, naltrexone, really cannot be subsumed under this title for numerous reasons.

Naltrexone is, in our opinion, ill-advised as an anti-opioid addiction medication, since it requires a person to be fully withdrawn from an opioid habit before taking it. This issue is, however, the least of the problems with this medication.

Besides having a high incidence of liver toxicity, the rate of medication compliance for the oral tablet form is exceedingly poor in withdrawn addicts, and for good reason. It usually takes the newly withdrawn addicted individual several days to figure out that naltrexone has *anhedonia* as one of its main side-effects. Anhedonia is simply an absolute inability to experience any kind of pleasure. It is thought that this occurs because naltrexone blocks both exogenous and endogenous opioids, and endogenous opioids are necessary for the experience of pleasure. Interestingly, anhedonia is not a side effect experienced by individuals addicted to alcohol who take naltrexone to relieve the urge to drink, but only in former opioid addicted individuals, probably indicating some long-term, permanent changes to the brains of opioid addicted individuals.

While there is a form of depot injection, i.e. long-lasting intramuscular naltrexone, abstinence rates with this form are still abysmal, as can be seen from studies of this dosage form in Russia; both of the following quotes are from Russian studies testing depot naltrexone, and the rates of relapse are still astonishing.

"*Opioid positive* urines at six months were *lowest* in the naltrexone implant group (*63%*), and higher in the oral naltrexone and placebo trials (87 and 86%, respectively)."

"Total abstinence measured as 100% opioid-free weeks in weeks 5 through 24 was 35.7% in the extended-release naltrexone group versus 22.6% in the placebo group." [1]

From *any* objective standpoint, 63% opioid positive urines at 6 months-out can only be considered a dismal failure of naltrexone to effectively stop continued opioid self-administration. Somewhat indicative of the cynicism with which the Russian government views opioid addiction, naltrexone is the only medication officially approved for use in the treatment of opioid addiction in that country. Without needle-exchanges and methadone and buprenorphine legally available, the Russian Federation, accordingly, has the highest proportion of illicit opioid addicts in the world (an unofficial tally has the number at about 2 million, out of a population of circa 195 million,) the vast majority of them already infected with hepatitis B, C, and HIV.

The American Society of Addiction Medicine, in a 2015 guidance statement, probably best summarized the minimal utility of naltrexone as an addiction medication.

"Oral naltrexone for the treatment of opioid use disorder is often adversely affected by poor medication adherence. Clinicians should reserve its use for patients who would be able to comply with specialized techniques to enhance their adherence, for example, with observed dosing. Extended-release injectable naltrexone reduces, but does not eliminate, issues with medication adherence." [3]

Buprenorphine, usually in some fixed combination with naloxone, is a partial opioid agonist that can have value in treating opioid addicted individuals, however, since it is much newer and less widely researched than methadone, we have chosen to leave it out of this book. There are other drawbacks and contraindications to buprenorphine.

Methadone, by contrast, can be used in any and every opioid addicted individual with success, provided that there is a willingness to do whatever is necessary to become stabilized on it. The entire methadone dispensing system in the U.S., in the form of specialized Opioid Treatment Program (OTP) clinics, is extremely regulated and in no way intersects with the regular healthcare system. This factor is only one of a number of weaknesses concerning methadone service delivery in this country, and it is discussed in greater detail in several chapters of this book.

It is our sincerest hope that this book will be but the first of many public-education campaigns regarding methadone maintenance treatment (MMT) as the best, and certainly by far most effective treatment modalities for opioid addiction. [8] As it now stands, the stigma regarding MMT is so great that precisely the people who could benefit from it most are also avoiding it the most, for a mixed bag of stigmatized reasons, which will also be elaborated upon and dealt with in subsequent chapters.

It can not go without saying that methadone is but one of a number of opioid agonist medications that have utility in medication assisted treatment (MAT,) especially maintenance. Pharmacologically speaking, for example, levorphanol (Levo-Dromoran) comes in a close second after methadone in terms of its potential utility as a treatment medicine. Whether or not this enters the MAT fold, particularly in the U.S., remains very much an open question. [4] Actual implementation of other opioid agonists besides methadone and buprenorphine would face an uphill battle considering how rigidly opioid treatment programs (OTPs) are regulated in the U.S., and how firmly ensconced these regulations are, but further discussion of this is beyond the scope of this book. (see Appendix I)

One final thought before we proceed. Throughout the long march of human history, it has been something of a given that most anyone who was too different, or stood out from the crowd just a bit too much, was either quickly beaten back into conformity or socially ostracized. In the 21st Century, we like to *consider ourselves civilized*, and when we look back at the many civil-right movements of the 1960's and 1970's, there is much that we can be proud of. No longer is it socially acceptable to disparage and discriminate against people of color, homosexuals, the disabled, and trans-gender individuals, and we are a better, stronger nation for it.

There is, however, still no social prohibition (not to mention inhibition) against discrimination and disparagement of the contemporary addict. As a rule, across the U.S., opioid addicts have died undergoing agonizing with-drawal in jails and prisons, disallowed from being properly medicated for their addictions. This is not conjecture: It is such an *unrecognized epidemic* that this book has a whole chapter dedicated to this most fundamental of human-rights violations – the right of any citizen to continued life, not premature death simply because that person is grotesquely and unfairly stigmatized. These jailhouse deaths are barely acknowledged by the main-stream media as being in any way problematic, and they have not yet hit the courts as *clear cases* of "cruel and unusual punishment."

We would do well to recognize this current state-of-affairs for what it is: *The last remaining civil rights frontier in the United States*, the right of addicted individuals to live a life unencumbered by relentless bigotry and persecution. Lest someone take offense at the use of the word persecution, they should quickly be reminded that some 74% of all healthcare providers endorse *very negative* prejudices about opioid addicts, and if a human being cannot find refuge from discrimination even within the walls of a hospital, then they are guaranteed to be subject to bigotry almost everywhere else.

The ugly reality is that no 21st Century American citizen is placed lower on the social totem-pole than the proverbial "drug addict." In the year 2020, this should be entirely unacceptable, and part of the goal of this book is to begin chipping away at these old prejudices and false assumptions. Let us begin by bringing the opioid-addicted back into the social-fold.

"Because there is no glory in illness. There is no meaning to it. There is no honor in dying of."

— John Green, The Fault in Our Stars

"I seem to myself, as in a dream, An accidental guest in this dreadful body."

— Anna Akhmatova, The Complete Poems of Anna Akhmatova

"Here I am trying to live, or rather, I am trying to teach the death within me how to live."

— Jean Cocteau

"In this country, don't forget, a habit is no damn private hell. There's no solitary confinement outside of jail. A habit is hell for those you love. And in this country, it's the worst kind of hell for those who love you."

— Billie Holiday, Lady Sings the Blues

"I used to condemn junkies, like they could get off the stuff if they really wanted to, and that is just as stupid as saying, "You could grow eyes in the back of your head if you really wanted to."

— Philip K. Dick, Philip K. Dick: The Last Interview
and Other Conversations

"Half a truth is often a great lie."

— Benjamin Franklin

1

IT'S NOT YOUR FAULT: THE FUTILITY OF PLACING "BLAME"

One of the most important themes that will be revisited over and over again in this book will be the importance of the opioid addicted individual understanding that, irrespective of the stigma and preconceived notions that greater society may have about addiction in general, opioid addiction is no ones fault, and most certainly not that of addicted individuals themselves.

Ascribing blame to an individual who has developed an addiction to drugs is akin to ascribing a nefarious motive to someone who has contracted a deadly virus; because a virus is by its very nature inanimate, attempting to attach a motive to its host is beyond a moot point. In the final analysis, we find it counterproductive to ascribe words such as "evil" to ultimately inanimate chemicals like drugs, for drugs have no effect until they enter a living organism, and in fact require that organism's machinery to produce their effects, not at all unlike a virus. Using this analogy, it is important to bear in mind that the vast majority of viruses are not pathogenic to humans, or "bad." They are, in fact, necessary for the process of evolution (horizontal gene transfer) and serve a crucial niche function in marine microbiology via a process known as the viral shunt, among other positive functions in biology.

Opioid addiction is a complex, multi-factorial disease that is the result of a conglomeration of factors that aggregate together in one person to produce the phenomenon. [6,7,8] These factors include, but are not limited to, ones genetics, environment, life stressors and, according to arguably the most consequentially important large-scale public health study to emerge in decades, a phenomenon known as Adverse Childhood Experiences (ACE's.) [7]

Because these factors are so varied in their origin and distribution, we refer to opioid addiction, and addiction in general, as being a biopsychosocial illness. This is because the effects of one factor, like possessing a genetic predisposition, are difficult to tease apart from other contributing factors like having a mentally ill parent, being a victim of childhood neglect, or coming from an impoverished household, among other things.

Nevertheless, all other things being equal, some factors undoubtedly play a more central role than do others. At the top of the list would be possessing a genetic predisposition, for without that genetic predisposition, addiction itself will not take hold. As to the precise nature of what the predisposing factors may all be, they have not yet been established; however, it has become exceedingly clear to researchers over the past two decades that a genetic predisposition is necessary in order for an individual to go on and develop an opioid addiction. [5]

A note on language and its power to both stigmatize and redeem. The reader will note that in this book, we intentionally avoid using words such as "clean," "dirty," "addict," and "junkie," unless they are context dependent and appropriate because these words have traditionally been used as weapons against opioid addicted individuals who are, in the final analysis, both equally human and equally deserving of dignity and respect. It would behoove the reader to remind himself or herself that language can be a powerful tool for both good and evil.

The fact that the term "addict" is used so freely by members of both the medical profession and the criminal justice system – and frankly, even by addicted individual themselves – attests to how powerful this word has become as a moniker that serves to both identify afflicted individuals *and* as a pejorative with which to condemn them. We can begin to change that today.

Opioid addiction does not happen in a vacuum. There are other risk factors besides the fundamental genetic vulnerability that come into play, and the weight that must be ascribed to these other factors should be considered to be at least as much as genetics, for just as without genetics, there would be no addiction, without the environment interacting with those genetics, there wouldn't be addiction. Later on, we will discuss the genetics and epigenetics of opioid addiction, but for now, let us discuss some of the other factors that come into play.

From 1995 to 1997, over 17,000 people were recruited into one of the most extensive longitudinal health studies in the U.S. that looked into the effects of adverse childhood experiences (ACE's) on public health. Because of the epidemiological value of the data, the study was conducted by the Kaiser Permanente HMO and the Centers for Disease Control, and what has come out of their findings is genuinely stunning and should serve as a societal wake-up call.

It absolutely bears mentioning that this study, which is still ongoing in different locales in the U.S., had its origins in an apparent medical mystery: in 1985, a physician by the name of Vincent Felitti found himself at a loss as to why more than half of the patients enrolled at his obesity clinic in San Diego were dropping out of the program every year for five years straight, even though they were all successfully losing substantial amounts of weight. It was as if just as they were making significant progress in achieving their weight loss goals, they dropped out.

Their withdrawal so puzzled Dr. Felitti that he decided to call in a couple of hundred of the former patients for an exit interview. Many interviews were conducted in which he discovered nothing that could explain these baffling results, until one day, while interviewing a female patient, he misspoke. While he had wanted to ask how old a woman had been during her first sexual encounter, he accidentally asked how much she weighed during her first sexual experience. The answer he received floored him: The woman he was interviewing broke down and spoke of incest she endured at the hands of her father when she was just four years old and all of forty pounds.

Over the next few days, as he began to ask the question of the other dropouts, he found something astonishing – nearly every study participant reported similar trauma during childhood. Ever the good scientist and to ensure that he was not introducing any unconscious bias into the interviews, he asked other colleagues to conduct the rest of the interviews. To his astonishment, they all reported the same results – serious childhood trauma in the obesity clinic dropout group.

Dr. Felitti was so intrigued by what he found that he became one of the principal investigators in the ACE's Study, along with a physician by the name of Robert Anda. They and their colleagues have been following 17,000 members of the Kaiser Permanente health insurance organization since 1995, collecting longitudinal data on their relative health and morbidity. One must bear in mind that they first gave each of these patients a ten-item questionnaire (Appendix II) as they initially enrolled in the study between 1995 and 1997, then they simply followed the medical data on each subject. [9,10]

"This was the first time that researchers had looked at the effects of several types of trauma, rather than the consequences of just one. What the data revealed was just mind-boggling. I wept. I saw how much people had suffered, and I wept." Robert F. Anda, M.D., M.S. [9]

"ACEs have created a chronic public health disaster." Robert Anda, M.D., M.S. [10]

What researchers found has been truly earth-shattering in its consequences. For each ACE an individual accumulated, there was a corresponding increase in morbidity and mortality *from all causes*, with the degree of morbidity and mortality being easily predicted *decades ahead of time* just by the relative accumulation of Adverse Childhood Experiences. There is truly no specialty of medicine that is exempted from these findings, and that includes opioid addiction treatment. [7,9]

An ACE score of four makes one ten times as likely to inject drugs, seven times as likely to develop alcoholism, twelve times more likely to attempt suicide, and 32 times more likely to be labeled with a behavioral or cognitive problem than a child with no ACEs. The numbers from the study are truly stunning, especially considering that even when the children were removed from the toxic environment, the lasting damage had been done. [9]

What requires mentioning at this point is that a high ACE score neither predestines an individual into becoming an opioid addict nor causes one to develop a mental illness; as such, not all people with traumatic childhoods come out for the worse. There is such a thing known as resilience. What can probably best be said about resilience among trauma survivors is that it, too, is most likely the luck of the genetic draw, to use a phrase. [11]

In the late 1970s at Simon Fraser University in British Columbia, a psychologist by the name of Bruce Alexander did some hard thinking followed by experimentation regarding opioid addiction and its causes. His experiment was called Rat Park (rats were his subjects), and the crucial result that he came up with was that animals do not automatically become addicted to opioids just because opioids are present in the environment. He found that something else was necessary to create addiction-like behavior in the rats – a lack of social connection and a poor, unenriched environment.

Since his paper appeared in 1978, Rat Park lost its funding from Simon Fraser University, and the results have been slightly modified from the original paper. It turns out that genetics also play a significant role in which individual rats become addicted to opioids. Just as there are strains of rats resistant to opioid addiction, so too are there strains of rats that are more susceptible to develop addiction. [5]

This has significant implications for the genesis of human opioid addiction. As has been mentioned before, the development of opioid addiction does not happen in a vacuum. There have to be vulnerable individuals with certain environmental constraints. This goes a long way toward explaining why the vast majority of people can take or leave opioids, with only a small minority who go on to develop severe addiction.

In light of the Rat Park experiment, one begins to understand why, in some respects, opioid addiction is also disease of loneliness. Lack of social connection is a primary cause of addiction, and then later becomes one of the results of opioid addiction as social ostracism in response to the addiction creeps in. For someone who is not already traumatized, a lack of social connection can be inconsequential, at best. For someone who is already coming to the scene with serious trauma, a lack of social connection can be the nail in the proverbial coffin.

The aforementioned causes of opioid addiction are an enormous part of the whole picture, but they do not explain everything.

One of the issues that has puzzled researchers over the decades is why individuals no longer physically addicted to opioids relapse, even after having been abstinent and in recovery for long periods of time. One hint lies in the particular tenacity of opioid addiction. There is strong evidence that opioid use by vulnerable individuals induces long-term, epigenetic changes in some regions of the brain that are crucial for motivation and goal-directed behavior. We will look at some of these changes in later chapters.

The sheer *tenacity* of severe opioid addiction is the reason why any traditional negative consequences of use have *no effect* on the addicted individual's likelihood for relapse, whether they have been abstinent for one day, one year, or one decade. Even though it has been known for at least 100 years that opioid addiction has the highest rates of recidivism, our criminal justice system and healthcare system as a whole have been largely ignorant of this. The abysmal recovery rates for abstinent opioid addicted individuals have served as a living and dying testimony to this reality.

The tremendous number of myths, the brutality of the stigma, the lack of up-to-date useful information, and the lack of more widespread availability of clinics to serve this patient population have all served as additional incentives for the examination of this issue.

Some readers may wonder why the emphasis is essentially entirely focused on methadone, with little to no reference to buprenorphine (Suboxone). The answer is quite straightforward: Suboxone, and its other proprietary and generic versions, is still *very*, very expensive when compared with methadone, and the long-term data on Suboxone maintenance is not nearly as robust as is the data on MMT. [8]

Adding to the complications, fewer and fewer insurers are covering Suboxone/buprenorphine treatment, making it less and less accessible to the very people who would benefit from it. [12] For this reason, the choice for focusing on methadone was made, as methadone is the first opioid agonist treatment ever to become widespread, over many decades, and in many countries throughout the world.

Another important reason why Suboxone/buprenorphine is not addressed in this book is for the simple reason that Suboxone is not effective for everyone with an opioid addiction, particularly if one happens to have a "heavy," long-standing addiction, as Suboxone may even put one into a state of withdrawal. Stated another way, methadone will work for anyone with an opioid addiction whereas Suboxone will only work in a particular sub-group of patients, usually those younger and less experienced with opioids.

Looking at the success of well-administered MMT, it is the cheapest and most effective treatment modality available for opioid addiction disorder. [8,29] The costs of other, non-evidence-based treatment modalities can also be measured in real dollars and cents, but these pale in comparison to the human and societal cost of such "treatments." With abstinence-based treatments, overdoses, both fatal and non-fatal, are just a "normal" part of the picture. We consider this to be an unacceptable outcome in any case, as every human being has the right to live another day. Let us not, in our haste, throw the baby out with the bath-water.

2

BENZODIAZEPINES

While the primary focus of this book is on methadone as a medication and treatment for opioid addiction, we would be remiss not to discuss the issue of concurrent benzodiazepine use with either methadone or buprenorphine therapy.

The main reason why benzodiazepines are important enough to warrant a separate chapter is because a significant number of Methadone Maintenance Treatment (MMT) patients have coexisting psychiatric diagnoses, with anxiety and bipolar disorder being among the most common ones. It is, in fact, somewhat unusual to find an MMT patient who has not required or does not currently require benzodiazepines. This, of course, in the current atmosphere of prosecution and persecution, can present many problems for recovering MMT patients, such as outside physicians insisting upon discontinuation of the benzodiazepine irrespective of medical necessity. [13,16]

Much has been said and written about the dangers and contraindications of benzodiazepine and opioid co-prescription, particularly with respect to the fact that the combination of medications can have an increased respiratory depressant effect in patients. [14] While it is true that there have been many opioid overdoses wherein benzodiazepines have been detected, upon closer inspection, it can be impossible to discern or ferret out what proportion of those overdoses were actually caused by a synergistic interaction between the benzodiazepine present and the opioid involved.

This is where statistics can become very deceiving because while opioid overdoses have increased, so too have opioid overdoses with benzodiazepines, and it is difficult to eliminate confounding factors such as what the acute dosage of the benzodiazepine actually was, whether it was legitimately prescribed, whether alcohol played a synergistic role with both medications, etc. This is due to the fact that very often only qualitative analysis of intoxicants present is done with autopsy drug panels. It is only the absolute presence of a substance that is established in such reports, making the relative contribution of various intoxicants to the persons' death rather opaque.

For individuals who have never had to deal with severe anxiety problems, this all might seem superfluous. However, for a good proportion of MMT patients, benzodiazepines can genuinely make an important and positive difference in their daily quality of life, and that is why it is so important for physicians not to succumb to "junkie" stereotypes when it comes to this particular patient population. In point of fact, Generalized Anxiety Disorder (GAD) can render sufferers incapable of even leaving their homes, and these same individuals sometimes must be admitted to Emergency Rooms due to cardiac symptoms brought about by panic attacks that are a common feature of GAD.

There is currently much controversy among physicians and clinical workers regarding this issue, but it must be stated that oftentimes emotion and anecdotal observations seem to trump reason and medically well-established guidelines. Irrespective of current prescribing trends, the reality is that there are no absolute contraindications to the co-prescription of benzodiazepines with opioids, only relative contraindications or as determined by the individual patient's medical history (such as in the presence of C.O.P.D, asthma, alcoholism, delirium, etc.). With respect to this matter, the FDA has recently reaffirmed that there are no absolute contraindications to coadministration. [13-16]

Ideally speaking, whether or not MMT patients should receive benzodiazepines must be left up to the physician in consultation with the patient and the patient's other treating physicians, not applied as a one-size-fits-all blanket policy, which is unfortunately how this has begun to take place all too frequently in recent years. [15]

That there are MMT facilities with a "zero-tolerance" stance on benzodiazepines is a current reality, with other facilities falling somewhere further up along the benzodiazepine tolerance continuum. Because there is no evidence-based codification within the federal guidelines regarding concurrent benzodiazepine prescription in the context of MMT, this is a rather typical example of each clinic operating as an island unto itself, with the patient being on the losing end of this biopsychosocial opacity.

Neglecting to use benzodiazepines in MMT patients who require them can present serious complications in their treatment and jeopardize their recovery, since anxiety is a disorder that is very frequently self-medicated, meaning that if the patient cannot legitimately obtain benzodiazepines, they will potentially seek to obtain them in some other manner or substitute them with even more dangerous drugs. The most commonly used substitute is alcohol, which poses a tremendous problem specifically for methadone maintenance treatment patients because alcohol accelerates the rate of metabolism or the rate at which the liver removes methadone from the body, which of course leads to early symptoms of withdrawal in between dosing, which in turn further renders the patient at risk of relapsing.

In the interest of a comprehensive review of this topic, it remains to be said that there are some MMT patients who simply abuse benzodiazepines, whether they receive them legitimately and for a medical indication or not. This reality not only shouldn't be denied, but must be looked squarely in the eye. For whatever reason, there will always be a percentage of MAT patients who abuse benzodiazepines given the chance. [17]

The important thing to remember is that it is crucial for a treating physician to not make an absolute judgment on their administration without having further evidence of any improprieties. This evidence could present itself in several ways, probably most commonly in seeing patients at an MMT clinic who present as clearly intoxicated, as evidenced by slurred speech, slowed thought processes, and "nodding", which simply looks like the patient is repeatedly and periodically falling asleep, only to reawaken with a start before nodding off again. [17]

Another common presentation is the presence of ataxia, which is simply an unsteady gait as the person attempts to walk forward. In this respect, some of these symptoms slightly resemble public drunkenness. That all patients must be dealt with on a case-by-case basis, in order to eliminate the possibility of withdrawing lifesaving and necessary medication from a patient who needs it, must become a part of the standard protocol at all MMT clinics, and not just left to the personal whims of individual clinic providers. [13]

Another critical point regarding benzodiazepine use in this patient population is that not all benzodiazepines work equally well together with methadone or buprenorphine. In particular, benzodiazepines such as Xanax (alprazolam,) Ativan (lorazepam,) Restoril (temazepam,) and Halcion (triazolam) can all cause greatly synergistic sedation with the opioid agonist the MMT patient is taking. This interaction can lead to a patient looking intoxicated even though they may be on a regimented and prescribed dose of that benzodiazepine and at an appropriate dose of methadone or buprenorphine.

Experience has shown that Klonopin (clonazepam) is perhaps the most ideal benzodiazepine for MMT patients since it does not cause excessive additive sedation with the opioid agonist. [138] Less is known about the interaction of opioid agonists with the older benzodiazepines such as Valium (diazepam,) Librium (chlordiazepoxide,) and Tranxene (clorazepate dipotassium,) for example.

Having now addressed some of the potential problems, it is important at this juncture to note that in those MMT patients who are taking their legitimately prescribed benzodiazepines as directed, when done properly, there should be no external signs that this combination is, in fact, being used. Stated another way, it must be difficult, if not impossible, to distinguish the so-called pure agonist patient from the agonist plus benzodiazepine patient. Once again, it must be emphasized that the circumstances and medication must be appropriately paired for a good outcome, but as has been said before, benzodiazepines can and do play a vital role in the recovery and maintenance of opioid addicted individuals on MMT.

One final word of caution. As you read the chapter on the stigmatization and marginalization of addicted individuals you will be made aware of what you are up against with respect to the medical profession providing benzodiazepines for MMT patients, and it is not insignificant. Most members of the medical profession, when guaranteed anonymity, endorse very negative views about opioid addicted patients, be they in MMT or not. [18,19]

3

The Peculiar History of Methadone: Addiction Treatment in the U.S. before Methadone and Where We are Today

"Drug users have had to overcome decades of silencing and incarceration to claim their right to health care and public health protection." [20]

Methadone was invented in Germany in the late 1930s by Gustav Ehrhart and Max Bockmuehl, researchers for Hoechst Farbenfabrik, a chemical company, and it was originally named Hoechst 10820 or Polamidon. As is so often the case in medicine, they arrived at its formulation serendipitously while searching for new anti-spasmodic drugs, never expecting that it would have any painkilling or opioid effects. After finding it to be an absolutely unremarkable antispasmodic agent in animal testing, it remained shelved for two to three years until Germany was fully entrenched in WWII.

It was at that point, when the Axis forces found themselves in the worst possible position to obtain the necessary morphine for their injured troops, that methadone came down from the shelf and enjoyed a brief stint as a morphine substitute on the battlefield. Doctors soon realized, however, that it could not be reliably used as such because after soldiers were given a course of methadone for battle wounds, they exhibited higher rates of dangerous side effects when compared with those which were seen with morphine administration. Of course, at this point in time, no one knew the particular pharmacological properties of methadone, and what turned out to create serious problems on the WWII battlefield later became properties that ideally suited methadone for opioid agonist therapy.

For the sake of brevity and as the saying goes, "to the victor go the spoils." After the détente, the United States obtained ownership of methadone's patent for the bargain basement price of one dollar. Eli Lilly of Indianapolis was the initial beneficiary, but they too soon found themselves in a similar quandary as Ehrhart and Bockmuehl in that here they had a full mu-opioid agonist (see Glossary) on their hands, which at the time was among the very first synthetic opioid agonists in the world, but which they soon found possessed no real commercial value because of the adverse effects of longer-term administration in patients.

These adverse effects became apparent within three to four days after administration and were evidenced, most clearly, by a deepening depression of the central nervous system. Patients were becoming increasingly opioid intoxicated, with this intoxication being manifested by decreased breathing and heart rates. This depressant effect is due to the fact that human beings have an abundance of opioid receptors in the brain stem which control the basic autonomic functions of the body, and though methadone has a half-life of approximately 24-30 hours in most people, its analgesic effects last only 6 hours, which can result in a dangerous accumulation of methadone in a neophyte's body as repeated doses for pain are administered. [22]

Methadone was then reshelved at Elly Lilly's headquarters and though they initially found almost no commercial use for methadone, Eli Lilly did utilize the methadone structural "scaffolding" as something that could be chemically tweaked for other useful drug discoveries. Darvon (propoxyphene Hcl) is one example and, though successfully marketed for a half a century before being unceremoniously discontinued in 2010 for its potential to cause deadly heart rhythm problems, was a very commercially lucrative derivative of methadone.

In the United States, between the years of the 1930s through the 1960s, there was a steadily rising tide of opiate addiction developing in the nation's urban areas. As the reasons for this phenomenon are multi-factorial, we will only touch upon the two most salient ones here. A confluence of events took place in the United States which essentially created the archetype of the modern "junkie." First and foremost, America had opioid addicted individuals at the turn of the last century because access to opium, morphine, heroin, and cocaine was possible for anyone who walked into a pharmacy at the time. As hard as it may be to imagine, all of these drugs were available over the counter for very reasonable prices. A point that is rarely made, not unsurprisingly given the current hysteria, is *how few opioid addicted individuals there were considering this level of accessibility.* [20]

The Prohibition of these drugs came in the form of the 1914 Harrison Narcotics Act, which made the drugs prescription only, and it was enthusiastically received by all manner of "Vice Commissions," which were popular at the time because even smaller cities were beginning to have well-known neighborhoods, referred to as "Vice Districts," which were occupied by opium dens and brothels, bars and pool-halls.

The predominant thinking at the time was that if all of the current vices were prohibited from legally operating, they would quickly disappear and all would be well again. The anti-vice movement itself was the complex result of the influence of the religious remnants of the Temperance Movement, which viewed stoically enduring physical pain as a virtuous part of God's plan, as well as from the vestiges of Puritanism that held that to consume anything that even remotely produced carnal pleasure was to indulge in the sinful act of hedonism. [20]

Epidemiologically speaking, people who had become truly addicted to these perfectly legal pain relievers, many of them war veterans, eventually found themselves at the mercy of an increasingly draconian national policy towards opium and opium derivatives, and thus could no longer obtain their needed drug legally.

What the anti-vice crowd and their legislative backers never came to fully understand was that severe opioid addiction was *incurable and chronic in nature.* Oddly enough, over one hundred years later, this misunderstanding still pervades the conventional wisdom on opioid addiction.

It was at this point that the criminal element, whose infrastructure rapidly developed and became entrenched as a result of the first Prohibition (Harrison Narcotics Act, 1914), stepped in to fill the growing black market need for morphine, and increasingly heroin. At that time, those were the drugs of choice, since the militarization that we know of as the War on Drugs had not yet begun, and widespread alternatives to these opioids had not yet been developed.

For a short time after 1914, the federal government allowed physicians who worked in specialized clinics to prescribe morphine for addicts, but this only lasted until 1930 when the Bureau of Narcotics shuttered these clinics even though they were fully legal under the act. In the process, thousands of physicians were ruthlessly persecuted and prosecuted by the criminal courts. So, effectively, after 1930, the entire market for opioids opened wide for criminal exploitation, since no physicians would knowingly continue to prescribe opioids for an addicted individual. [20,23]

One of the solutions for a desperately addicted individual at that time was to travel to an institution in Lexington, Kentucky, called "The Narcotic Farm." The Farm was a combination prison/rehabilitation and research center owned by the State of Kentucky and overseen by what was known at the time as the Bureau of Narcotics and Dangerous Drugs (the BNDD). It opened in 1935 in Kentucky's rural countryside, and it accepted addicted individuals who arrived from all over the United States. Roughly two-thirds of its residents were considered voluntary patients and the remainder were sentenced to be there in lieu of potentially lengthy prison sentences for simple possession. [20, 23]

There, at the addicted individual's request and the doctor's proviso, the opioid addicted individual would reach his arm out of his locked cell and receive a daily, but gradually decreasing dose of morphine, which was oftentimes grossly inadequate to satisfy his requirement given the tolerance level he likely arrived with, but which was designed to "cure" him of his addiction by tapering him off the drug incrementally. This meager dose provided the addicted individual a brief period of relief, and then withdrawal would re-ensue. The Narcotic Farm's "success" rate at helping addicted individuals recover from their opiate addiction was reportedly 10%.

Knowing what we know today about the chronic and relapsing nature of this disease, that number is, at best, questionable. [20]

The consequences of The Farm's failures resulted in both predictable relapse rates and deepening addiction, with neither treatment nor cure to resolve them. The implications were dire for Americans with opioid addiction, who were forced to battle the constant cravings and survive the inevitable withdrawal syndrome, and for whom The Farm's failure was most acutely felt.

In 1974, The Farm was closed and redesignated as a federal prison. That it was closed only a few years after the introduction of methadone maintenance treatment in America is more than just coincidence. The powers-that-be experienced a paradigm shift in terms of the way they viewed opioid addiction and its treatment, a shift entirely due to the pioneering work of Dr.'s Vincent Dole and Marie Nyswander. Also painfully clear is that this paradigm shift was minimal and subject to many arbitrary changes over the ensuing years, as we see in both the extremely heterogeneous patchwork of MMT clinics in the States today and in the antiquated federal codes that regulate them. (Refer to chapters 8, 16, and Appendix I)

Although criminality and opioid addiction have historically been considered to be two sides of the same coin, nothing could be further from the truth. Addicted individuals will commit crimes in order to support their very expensive illness, which itself is a direct result of the prohibition of opioid possession by non-medical personnel. *Were it not illegal to be an opioid addicted individual, there would be no drug-related crime.* [20]

Evidence in support of this view has been found in study after study of people receiving medically assisted treatment (MAT). Opioid agonist therapy, be it with methadone, buprenorphine, heroin (which is legal in Switzerland) or any other agonist, vastly reduces the crime generally associated with opioid addiction. [24]

The reality of MMT, particularly regarding its effectiveness, is undeniable and runs completely contrary to all of the negative mythology that has sprouted up around it like a kudzu vine. With over 50 years of documented, evidence-based experience with MMT in the real world setting, this is the only treatment modality proven to work. [8, 24, 27, 40-42]

To be clear, by stressing MMT's efficacy, we are referring to its ability to keep opioid addicts in recovery, away from potential relapse and alive. As can be seen from the abysmal relapse rates of addicted individuals who have attempted to "kick" their addiction without medical assistance, these benchmarks can be tall orders to meet. [20, 23]

That having been said, the MMT system in the United States currently consists of approximately 1,200 clinics that are heterogeneous both in their geographic distribution as well as their individual treatment "philosophies." First, though it is difficult to establish objectively, approximately 1,200 clinics spread out over the North American continent seems like too few clinics for the current situation, where the number of patients, both potential and real, is seeing explosive growth. Considering the Substance Abuse and Mental Health Services Administrations (SAMHSA) national survey statistic of 2016, there were 2.1 million people addicted to prescription opioids or heroin. Doing the very rough math, that would come out to about 1600 patients per MMT clinic, bearing in mind that many clinics have a patient census of fewer than 1,000 individuals.

Secondly, and more importantly, the differing treatment philosophies between clinics can and do make for differing patient outcomes, as not all clinics are following the original Dole-Nyswander protocol. The importance of following the original protocol is so crucial precisely because Dole and Nyswander were so successful with the protocol that they had finally arrived at. Chief among their realizations was that proper, individualized dosing was the foundation for a robust recovery. Also among their findings was that higher dosages provided critical opioid blockade and vital craving suppression. [40-42]

Astonishingly, decades after Dole himself decried the notion of an upper limit on daily methadone dosage, too many clinics have treatment protocols that impose low dosage ceilings (generally, 100 mg/day or less) combined with a transitional notion of methadone's role in the recovery from opioid addiction. [41] These clinics view methadone as a means to an end, that end being the eventual achievement of abstinence from all forms of opioids, and in pursuit of this, they will actively encourage their patients to begin "tapering off" of the methadone after a period of time.

Not surprisingly, these kinds of clinics tend to operate like a revolving-door, with many patients constantly relapsing because their dose is just too low to be effective at preventing the return of cravings, which leads to the unacceptable sequelae that is typically involved in relapsing (illicit drug use, incarceration, overdosing, death, etc.). To say that this defeats the entire purpose of MMT is to state what should be obvious, but unfortunately isn't at too many MMT clinics across the country. [30, 31]

In one of the best studies to date that examines the effectiveness of "higher" dosages, Maxwell and Shinderman chose 164 patients who were not responding well to doses of up to 100 mg per day of methadone, as was evidenced by their extremely high rate of continued illicit opioid use (87%), and compared them to a randomly selected control group of patients receiving 69 mg per day of methadone on average (range: 10-100 mg).

The experimental, non-responder group were each titrated upwards to an individualized mean dose of 211 mg per day (range: 120-780 mg per day). The results they arrived at were undeniable: in the "high dose" experimental group, urines which tested positive for illicit opioids went down from 87% to 3%, whereas in the control group, positive urines only went down from 55% to 36%. In addition, the one-year or more retention rate at the clinic was 86% for the high dosage group, compared to 35% for the control group. [28]

Informally, every day across the U.S., MMT clinics that stay away from artificial, one-size-fits-all dosage limits enjoy tremendous success rates. People unfamiliar with MMT might ask themselves, "Well, then what's to limit every patient from just wanting more and more methadone?" The answer to this question lies in the very pharmacology of opioid addiction treatment with methadone. No matter how severe the opioid addiction, it is the exceptional patient who will keep trying to ramp-up their dose because once a sufficient opioid receptor occupancy in the brain is achieved for the right amount of time, cravings for more methadone or for any opioid ceases. In addition, each patient works closely with a prescribing physician who carefully observes, with a trained eye, for either opioid intoxication (too much) or opioid withdrawal (too little). Ideally, once a given patient reaches that dose that is right for their body, they are stabilized and ready to get on with their lives.

With an appropriate dose, an MMT patient is indistinguishable from your man-on-the-street, irrespective of how high or low the dose is that they may be taking. The key to emphasize once again is personalized dosing that is tailor-made for the individual's physiology, not a cookie-cutter dosing regimen. [41]

The dosage issue would not be an issue were it not for the aberrant practices of some misinformed clinicians and the grave consequences that these practices can exact on people's lives. The dosage problem is also reflective of another, related problem in the MMT field today. If there are clinicians out there who are satisfied with prescribing sub-optimal doses and getting the correspondingly adverse outcomes, it means that most of these physicians are not believing what their patients are conveying to them when it comes to breakthrough withdrawal symptoms, etc. This is tragic and it is reflective of a broken doctor-patient relationship and quite possibly the erroneous belief on the part of some clinicians that addicted individuals are constantly drug seeking when in the presence of a physician with a prescription pad. With a good clinical eye and thorough medical vetting, the patient should generally be given the benefit of the doubt when it comes to their subjective experience with the medication.

Why there are any of these low-dose, tapering clinics left in light of what is now known about effective MMT is a mystery whose answer can't be reassuring. [30] Let's change that.

4

WITHDRAWAL AND POST ACUTE WITHDRAWAL SYNDROME

It is reasonably safe to say that most neurotypicals (normal, unaddicted individuals) imagine the opioid addicted individual's sole motivation for continuing their use of opioids to be primarily rooted in the fear of the pain and torment of withdrawal. In reality, while fear of the pain of withdrawal plays a fractional role in one's motivation to continue use, it is by far and wide not the limiting factor. This is most clearly evidenced by the simple fact that opioid addicted individuals, while averse to withdrawing, nonetheless can manage to achieve full and complete withdrawal resulting in abstinence, if only in the most superficial sense of the word. [37]

The term superficial is used specifically because we must always bear in mind that beneath the one-dimensional caricature that is the archetypal "junkie," there really is an entire three dimensional human being, an individual with an entire history and life story. The reason why a superficial versus a deeper probing of addiction and addiction treatment can mean the difference between life and death for the addicted individual is because there is no true opioid addicted individual who hasn't been through complete withdrawal at least once. The numbers are very hard to come by because this is not the most desired population to seek grant money for, for the purposes of research and understanding, so we simply do not possess steady numbers.

However, for those unfamiliar with the physical and emotional processes of opioid withdrawal, a brief introduction follows. Withdrawal from opioids follows a predictable course and symptomatology, the severity of which can differ significantly depending on whether or not the person in question is genuinely an addicted individual or whether they are simply medically dependent. This distinction is important, and while we know of no studies that have examined this difference, we do know what has been seen anecdotally, over and over. For the true opioid addict, withdrawal from even a small "habit" can literally feel like torture, and brutal cravings are present throughout the process and especially after withdrawal has been achieved, whereas cravings are non-existent in the medically dependent person undergoing withdrawal. This distinction in the kind and degree of symptoms appears to help explain why most people have no trouble "walking away" from medical opioid use, whereas a small minority become rapidly and severely addicted. [20]

Another crucial distinction to be made, intertwined with those mentioned above, has to do with whether the opioids are being administered in the presence of serious physical pain, as opposed to just being used "recreationally." The presence of pain apparently confers some degree of protection, if you will, against the development of flagrant addiction, whereas conversely, the absence of physical pain is a risk factor for its development. Most importantly, and as will be repeatedly emphasized, though these phenomena are not absolute or 100% applicable to every scenario, they do provide a useful rule-of-thumb with which to interpret aggregate data.

So back to the process of withdrawing from opioids. For the genuinely addicted individual, withdrawal from opioids often begins with a vague feeling of uneasiness, progressing in its intensity until there is an agonizing crescendo of agitation, fear and anxiety that can rise to the level of panic. A cascade of influenza-like symptoms soon develops. The nose begins to run profusely, muscles will ache deeply, accompanied by alternating sweating and "cold flashes," gooseflesh and tremors. Added to this panoply, an adrenal storm then ensues. The addicted individual's heart rate, respiration rate and blood pressure may all rise to precipitously high levels. He will feel as though he is in the active process of dying, and his fears are not totally unfounded, because though deaths from withdrawal pale in comparison to those related to overdose, they may occur far more often than is officially acknowledged or reported. [38]

Most saliently, the addicted individual will experience an uncontrollable craving to quell these symptoms with the only substance that he knows can "fix" or alleviate his pain; more opioids. For this, he is blamed for possessing both a lack of willpower and poor moral fiber. [20] At this point in the process, the addicted individual may gradually begin to experience a sudden shut down of what were formerly voluntary bodily functions, such as defecation and urination. Nausea and vomiting may also occur. These manifestations of withdrawal may occur individually or simultaneously, and the particular constellation of symptoms experienced will depend upon the individual. Spontaneous ejaculation may also take place as the body, being entirely out of equilibrium, now furiously makes up for the activation of a previously suppressed hypothalamic-pituitary-gonadal axis. The sensitivity of the genitalia can, in fact, become so great that having any kind of undergarment on or even experiencing a passing breeze may generate an unpleasant orgasm. All of this frenzied physical agony that the addicted individual undergoes is indistinguishable to him from actual torture, so aversive is the body's response. It is not surprising then that suicidal ideation, and sometimes suicide itself, is a common feature of this syndrome.

To stick a fork in it, the addicted individual is unable to seek refuge in sleep, as sleep becomes a literal impossibility. It is not uncommon for a heroin or morphine addicted individual in withdrawal to be unable to fall asleep for any amount of time for up to a week. If continued abstinence is self-imposed or forced upon him, his ability to sleep may be compromised for the weeks and months that follow. Indeed, the whole of his body's natural rhythms, which in addition to sleep include metabolism, sex drive, cardiovascular functioning, digestion and especially, an overall sense of wellbeing, can take anywhere between several months and up to years to fully regain equilibrium. [38]

All empirical observation of randomly chosen opioid addicts will quickly disabuse one of the notion that it is the actual "quitting" that is stopping them from ending their disease. This is somewhat analogous to the nicotine addict; the problem with nicotine addiction is not in the stopping of the habit: people quit all the time. Despite what you have just read, withdrawal is not the most difficult part of this process. The difficulty only really starts a short time after one's body has achieved a rough equilibrium (wherein one can sleep, not experience withdrawal signs, etc.), and the now formerly addicted individual finds that they have not been left in the same physiological state that they enjoyed before they became addicted to opioids, but have been permanently and irrevocably altered by the drug. [42]

It is crucial to point out that at this point it is not entirely clear if the subset of alterations and adaptations that occur during opioid use in addicted individuals occur to any degree in neurotypicals, or that they occur at all in that population, thereby indicating that they may very well be specific to the vulnerable individual. It is not enough to apply the algorithm drug plus person equals addict, it has to be drug plus vulnerable individual creates an "addict." In this respect, it is a multifactorial, biopsychosocial disease because one cannot tease apart these elements into separate domains and then treat them as if one component were entirely independent from the other components.

The attempt here is to paint a rough picture of how truly complex opioid addiction, in particular, is in a way that fast "soundbite," twitter-type explanations simply cannot replicate. They may make a statement about something or another, but they cannot capture the broader social, environmental and economic factors – not to mention the genetic vulnerabilities at work. The interplay between vulnerability and this expanded paradigm are what need to be explained. Post Acute Withdrawal Syndrome or PAWS is a good way of first simply explaining why some individuals can come out of a detox facility, ostensibly relieved of the "monkey" on their back and no longer physiologically dependent on the drug, only to reinstate use of the drug at some point thereafter.

PAWS is precisely what its eponymous title indicates, meaning that initial withdrawal is not the end of any kind of healing or the beginning of some anabolic process. PAWS is almost invariably a very large contributing factor to ultimate relapse. With the withdrawal syndrome no longer being present, the problem is that because of the PAWS phenomenon, the opioid addicted individuals attempts at abstinence are almost biologically impossible. This is the extant reality.

What often ends up happening is that early on in their addiction journey, opioid addicted individuals go through withdrawal and, even though they never feel "right" again after the opioid has cleared their system, the problem is that they appear to family members and friends as healthy, perhaps even healthier than ever. It is with this unwitting self-deception on the part of family and loved ones that the unfortunate continuation of addiction can be fostered and essentially become the "revolving door" phenomenon that is very familiar to a large percentage of opioid addicted individuals. This is due to the fact that the now withdrawn individual looks healthy and recovered even though this is not a reflection of their inner feeling state. Since family and friends cannot experience their loved one's inner reality, they will have expectations for behavior that the newly detoxed individual may quite simply be unable to meet. This exerts pressure on him to perform, and he will naturally experience substantial distress at the enormous dichotomy of his external appearance vs. his internal reality. The solution to resolve this dichotomy will nearly always be to seek out opioids.

A tragic, significant proportion of opioid addicted individuals simply go through the revolving door of intoxication, withdrawal, temporary abstinence, and right back through to relapse. The metaphor that comes to mind here is that of a dog chasing its own tail endlessly, and never being able to catch it.

To the uninitiated, PAWS is arguably at least as difficult as the acute withdrawal experience and in many cases even more difficult to endure, because it is arduous for the addicted individual to reconcile their non-opioid dependent status with the overwhelming dysphoria they now experience. This dysphoria can take many forms, but is most commonly characterized by low-grade depression, free-floating anxiety, and seemingly unrelenting anhedonia, which is the inability to experience any form of physical or emotional pleasure, which can leave the individual feeling dead inside. This feeling state is accompanied by protracted disturbances to ones inner, biological clock, which can render the individual physically exhausted from severe sleep disruption, up to and including total insomnia, which is the inability to sleep for periods that can last as long as weeks.

To cap PAWS off, the individual is left with a certain degree of residual autonomic nervous system instability that manifests itself in the form of hot flashes, cold sweats, feeling cold even though it is objectively warm, generalized tremors and a reduced appetite, which is only worsened by the anhedonia, as the addicted individual can no longer experience even the simplest gustatory pleasure. These symptoms may be accompanied by a plethora of other general discomforts and complaints, and they may abate spontaneously only to return full-force for reasons that are not entirely understood.

PAWS can set in anytime after the end of the acute withdrawal period and can last, depending upon the opioid one is withdrawing from as well as other factors, from weeks to several months and in severe cases, stretching into several years. PAWS exacts a terrible cost from the addicted individual attempting recovery precisely because it removes any and all ability to experience any kind of pleasure or emotive feeling. This anhedonia renders the now "clean" addicted individual searching for a way to relieve the intolerable state of psychic purgatory that the addiction creates, and it is the leading cause of relapse in opioid-free individuals. [41]

However, the reality of PAWS need not render an addicted individual committed to recovery hopeless. What *can* alleviate PAWS is methadone maintenance treatment. Methadone maintenance effectively eliminates the PAWS phenomenon. This makes sense on every level because methadone is a full opioid agonist. Administering methadone directly addresses the metabolic derangements which are characteristic of opioid withdrawal, both acute and post-acute. [8, 42]

To the reader who may be thinking that this is just substituting one addiction for another and that methadone merely postpones eventual withdrawal, it can be stated that this is no different from how exogenously administered insulin merely postpones eventual hyperglycemia, with all of its attendant sequelae. There is no effective difference between the two, except for the fact that diabetes is treated just like any other chronic illness, whereas opioid addiction is not.

For far too many decades, medical professionals have thrown their hands in the air and *suggested* 12-step, abstinence-based treatment modalities for opioid addiction, with absolutely no evidence-base whatsoever as to their efficacy, short or long-term. It should therefore come as little surprise that as long as abstinence is the only socially acceptable treatment protocol considered, the guaranteed most effective treatment for opioid addiction will remain hidden in plain sight. As is mentioned further along in this book, there are plenty of problems with how MMT is currently delivered, so this is an area rife for reform. Considering the staggering rate of opioid overdoses that occur every year in the United States (circa 47,000 per annum), the time for reform is inarguably overdue. [43]

Considering the intractable nature of severe opioid addiction and its currently exploding rate of occurrence, it has become a moral imperative that there be an evidence-based treatment modality such as MMT available to anyone who needs it, irrespective of ones ability to pay. [8] As it now stands, methadone maintenance remains the most cost-effective treatment available, and now is the time for the federal government to revisit vastly expanded funding for more clinics across the nation, not to mention an update to the federal regulations regarding the delivery of MMT for the 21st Century. (see Appendix I)

To the reader who may think that we as a nation are capable of doing so much better by this vastly under-served demographic, the humane consideration is a change of the old paradigm. Instead of communities fighting the Not In My Back Yard (NIMBY) battles over clinics that are present in their neighborhoods, why not have open dialogue take place between community representatives and medical professionals to allay fears and dispel myths?

Most neurotypicals would be shocked to learn how heterogeneous MMT clinic populations can be, and how much more they share similarities with these communities rather than differences. At this point it is important to remind the reader that the only thing that sets a recovering opioid addicted individual apart from a neurotypical person is that the former must take a medication every day in order to stay healthy...then again, many neurotypical people must also take a daily medication to stay healthy, for example, if they have hypertension, heart disease, an autoimmune disorder, etc.

The more that one thinks it through, the clearer it becomes that opioid addiction is just like any other chronic, incurable disease: medication must be taken for a lifetime, and there is the risk of relapse that attends noncompliance with medical advice. [41, 42]

As Vincent Dole so clearly saw during the course of his research, methadone patients who are stabilized continue to live their lives as if nothing adverse had ever happened. They go to work, to school, and take vacations with their kids just like everybody else. Perhaps the greatest irony lays in the fact that methadone maintenance treatment, when performed correctly, is the most successful treatment modality to treat opioid addiction to have come along in the last 55 years. [27]

The greatest tragedy is that while individuals who fail at MMT are familiar to most people, the individuals who succeed are familiar only to the fewest, precisely because of the chilling effect that stigma has on the willingness of patients to disclose their treatment status, especially and precisely when they are experiencing nothing but success. Can anyone blame the MMT patient for not wanting to tell a soul about their treatment status, considering everything we now know about the vicious ostracism experienced by patients who were less-than-careful about disclosing their status?

The frequent complaints that MMT "does not work" mainly come from a small but *very visible* subset of MMT patients who are not gaining the full benefits of well-practiced MMT, itself not infrequently the result of improper MMT protocols and rampant under-dosing.

The greatest tragedy that can befall an opioid addicted individual is not being able to access MMT, for logistical or financial reasons. MMT gives the opioid addicted individual a new chance at life, and that is the greatest gift that one person can give another. Having been proven as the gold standard in the treatment of opioid addiction, MMT has spent 50 years effectively on probation. It is time to expand treatment availability to all who might require it and to improve and modernize its administration. [29]

5

THE PIONEERS OF MODERN OPIOID ADDICTION TREATMENT

Vincent Dole and Marie Nyswander set out to find out how and why some people became addicted to opioids, and perhaps most importantly, how best to treat this condition. They arrived at the conclusion that opioid addiction, once fully entrenched in a vulnerable individual, is only survivable with what they called substitution therapy. The designation for MMT changed from substitution therapy to Opioid Agonist Therapy when it became clear that laypersons were confusing MMT with "substituting one addiction for another."

Vincent Dole was a physician who took a particular research interest in endocrinology and the disturbances of metabolism. In the early 1960s, he invited Dr. Marie Nyswander, a psychologist who specialized in the research of addictions, to join him in exploring his hypothesis that addiction was rooted in a metabolic disturbance in the brain. Towards that end, having already been familiar with the singularly unique pharmacology of methadone, they realized that it might be possible to provide an addicted individual an oral, daily dose of medication that would stave off not only withdrawal but the craving for opioids itself so that the affected individual could literally start focusing on something other than obtaining the next period of endocrine relief.

It must be noted that Dole and Nyswander were not able to proceed without running into serious difficulties with what was then known as the Federal

Bureau of Narcotics (FBN) division of the Treasury Department, the same agency that is now known as the DEA (Drug Enforcement Administration). It is no exaggeration to suggest that had Dole, in particular, been a more sheepish individual, MMT may never have seen the light of day. At the time, the disbelievers and naysayers were in an overwhelming majority where it counted most, in the federal government. The history books have only given the story of this harassment short shrift, so it bears retelling here; [44]

"In 1962, Vincent Dole and Marie Nyswander at Rockefeller University began planning clinical studies to use methadone with carefully selected narcotic addicts in New York City. Their research, which started in late 1963, and was first reported by Dole in 1965, demonstrated that methadone could be used to treat intractable heroin addicts by maintenance, not detoxification."

"Beginning in the mid-1960s, the findings of Dole, Nyswander and Mary Jeanne Kreek were reported in a number of papers (Dole, et al., 1966). As a result, many interested researchers and clinicians visited Rockefeller to learn about their treatment protocols. Annual conferences held from 1968 through 1971, and sponsored by the National Association for the Prevention of Addiction to Narcotics, resulted in the rapid dissemination of this research and the creation of a close professional network to promote the use of methadone in treating heroin addiction (Besteman interview)."

"Dole's planning in the mid-1960s included an assessment of the legal authority of Rockefeller University to conduct such research. Although Dole and Nyswander's studies provided the clinical demonstration of effectiveness, they were not done under an Investigational New Drug (IND) license, as FDA rules did not require one. Dole viewed the Treasury's Bureau of Narcotics (FBN) as the primary federal agency that might have regulatory authority over his proposed research, and the key question was whether research using methadone to maintain heroin addicts as part of a treatment program in New York City was within the domain of the professional practice of medicine or was another form of trafficking, as FBN had claimed with respect to the morphine clinics some 40 years earlier (Dole, 1989)."

"After extensive consultation with university lawyers and officials, Dole concluded that prior Supreme Court decisions did not bar the use of methadone in "in the course of professional treatment." The FBN view, however, was that maintenance of narcotic addiction with any narcotic drug fell outside the normal course of professional treatment. Dole recalls a visit by an FBN agent who informed him that he was breaking the law and that he would be put in jail. Dole challenged his visitor to have the agency sue him, a distinguished member of the faculty of Rockefeller University. Nonplussed, the agent left, only to return a short time later with the message that the research could be conducted, but only under the direction of the Bureau. Dole, secure in his knowledge of the limits of FBN authority, rejected this concession as well (telephone interview with Dr. Vincent Dole, December 1993). For roughly a five-year period, from 1965 through 1970, Dole's research went forward, harassed by the FBN, as Dole recalls, but without regulatory encumbrances." [44]

That methadone remains *officially stigmatized* is evidenced by the fact that by definition (and ensconced in law,) MMT clinics must be run separately from and outside of the regular healthcare system. Federal regulations mandate this. What is also by the regulations is the hypocritical double-standard regarding methadone which dictates that if it is to be used for addiction treatment, it must only be dispensed from one of the heavily regulated clinics, but if it is prescribed for pain, the prescription can be legally filled at any pharmacy.

Stated another way, opioid addicted individuals have been so stigmatized that they are kept as separate from "regular" patients as is possible, by federal statute. "A methadone patient is monitored more closely than a paroled murderer," said Dr. Edwin A. Salsitz, who runs the methadone program at Beth Israel Hospital in New York City. "Even someone who may be working has to be monitored because of regulations, and clinics themselves come up with regulations," Dr. Salsitz said. [45]

As a recent Institute of Medicine review concurred, "...the current policy puts too much emphasis on protecting society from methadone, and not enough on protecting society from the epidemic of addiction, violence, and infections that methadone can help reduce." [46]

Still, despite all the harassment by the FBN, Dole and Nyswander persisted, and countless people have them to thank for their lives because they remained steadfastly undeterred. Their research was sponsored by the Rockefeller Institute (now Rockefeller University) in New York City and ultimately rendered the discovery of MMT as an effective treatment for opioid addiction. Dr. Dole's hypothesis and idea, once subsequently fleshed out in the lab, proved to exceed his grandest expectations;

"Drug-seeking behavior, like theft, is observed after addiction is established and the narcotic drug has become euphorigenic. The question as to whether this abnormality in reaction stems from the fundamental weakness of character, or is a consequence of drug usage, is best studied when drug hunger is relieved. Patients on the methadone maintenance program, blockaded against the euphorigenic action of heroin, turn their energies to school, work and jobs. It would be easy for them to become passive, to live indefinitely on public support and claim that they had done enough in winning the fight against heroin. Why they do not yield to this temptation is unclear, but in general, they do not. Their struggles to become self-supporting members of the community should impress the critics who had considered them self-indulgent when drug-hungry addicts. When drug hunger is blocked without the production of narcotic effects, the drug-seeking behavior ends." [42]

This is why Dole and Nyswander's research was considered seminal and to this day is the gold standard protocol that skilled addiction specialists use to treat chronic opioid addiction. Opioid agonist therapy, a more general term for MMT, is the only treatment modality that can ensure the survival of the vast majority of addicts in the long term. Anything less allows the addicted individual to live on borrowed time, their eventual death from opioid overdose likely, if not assured.

The World Health Organization, a branch of the United Nations which is to the world what the CDC is to the United States, biannually issues a list that is known as the 100 Essential Medicines. What is meant by this is that there are minimal medications for a health system to have on hand, ones that are considered indispensable in the sustenance of life and the maintenance of health. On this list, methadone is contained under the rubric of "Medicines for Disorders due to Psychoactive Substance Use," as well us under "Opioid Analgesics." If the World Health Organization has long determined that methadone maintenance is the only proven, evidence-based effective medical treatment for opioid addiction in the last 50 years, medical professionals should sit up and take note. [47]

Ever since the advent of opioid agonist treatment via Methadone Maintenance Therapy, it holds the unique and singular distinction of being the most clinically studied, peer-reviewed, researched, published and successfully applied treatment modality of all other treatment modalities combined. A reasonable assumption can be drawn as to its efficacy. [32]

Given that all of the aforementioned information has been set in stone and relied upon for the past 50 years by *skilled treatment specialists*, the reader may ask himself why it is that these facts have escaped the consciousness of the general zeitgeist and, in point of fact, why it is all too often not even known to or accepted by addicted individuals themselves?

Anecdotal evidence suggests that a significant majority of addicts are given to conspiratorial thinking about methadone. It is not uncommon to hear addicted individuals emphatically state, "I'll be damned if I'm going to let big pharma make money off of my misery!" or "I'm not gonna stay on this "junk" forever!" or for them to attribute to clinic personnel nefarious motives that involve imagined personal vendettas, to develop persecution complexes, or to succumb to paranoid ideation. [138]

These deeply felt misperceptions are rooted in the fact that in 21st Century America, opioid addicted individuals have, through no fault of their own, simply internalized the vast number of negative messages, microaggressions and indignities that they experience on a daily basis because of the brutal stigmatization and discrimination their society inflicts upon them. It can be psychologically overwhelming to navigate the rough seas of addiction and societal scorn without drowning in a sea of negative, often unstated messages. [20]

What doesn't help to reduce this conspiratorial thinking is the fact that so many of todays MMT clinics are set up like a proverbial circus-hoop jump circuit. In order to continue being a patient in good standing, one is required to perform x, y, and z, actions which at times appear wholly arbitrary and petty, whether they are or not. Most people eventually want as little contact with their MMT provider as is possible, and yet there are still far too many clinics that have unrealistic rules which call for more contact than long-term patients are comfortable with. (see Appendix I)

Why Methadone Maintenance Treatment is so irrationally stigmatized when we think nothing of sitting at the local pancake house and seeing an obese patron injecting insulin after an unhealthy meal, or passing by an individual on the street with nicotine-stained fingers who is suffering from COPD, with their oxygen tank slung over their shoulder, sheds light on the fact that there are so many "lifestyle" diseases that require *daily dependence on a medication*, the only difference being that they are either socially acceptable or tolerated, while maintenance treatment for opioid addiction is not. It is arbitrarily unfair. How is the overweight pancake house patron, whose life depends on the daily administration of a drug through a hypodermic needle, so vastly different from the addicted individual, whose disease large portions of society refuse to even acknowledge as an actual disease?

For those who think a stint in the criminal justice system is just what is needed to "cure" any addicted individual, I would point to the staggering relapse and overdose rates of just-released inmates. Clearly, part of what is needed here is the presence of Medication Assisted Treatment (MAT) in jails and prisons, which is now the absolute exception in the U.S., even though these in-jail programs have been proven over and over again to greatly reduce morbidity and mortality for recently discharged opioid addicted individuals. What is currently the great shame of the U.S. is that addicted individuals are forced to withdraw "cold-turkey" when they arrive in jail, a policy which has resulted in too many jailhouse deaths across the nation, and corresponding lawsuits for wrongful deaths. (see Chapter 14)

The mentality that addicted individuals can be punished into abstinence is an indisputable fallacy, long known to physicians, psychologists and behaviorists, but not to the criminal justice system or the public at large. The "punishment" for an individual addicted to opioids is that they have irrevocably developed a brutal disease that is not even acknowledged as such by a substantial part of the population. The disease is a life sentence in and of itself; its walls are insurmountable, its course is largely fixed and unalterable, and like every other chronic life long illness, it is best treated and managed outside of prison walls as there is no amount of pain or deterrence that will stop an addicted individual from using again (see Chapters 6, 14 & 15).

Why and how is irrelevant, what is crucial to realize is that this is axiomatic for severely opioid addicted individuals. Moreover, the illicit use of opioids is always tied to a steep risk of accidental overdose.

"What a wonderful world it would be if the simplistic view were accurate: that human beings need only negative consequences to teach them hard lessons. Then any number of fast food franchises would be tickets to bankruptcy, the TV room would be an empty spot in our homes and the Portland Hotel [ed. Note: a S.R.O. for addicted individuals in Vancouver, B.C.] could reinvent itself as something more lucrative: perhaps a luxury housing unit with Mediterranean pretensions." [27]

There is a vast gulf separating the general public's understanding of what opioid addiction is and what it is not. The metastasizing opioid epidemic, which is finally considered a cause worthy of the public's attention and the government's compassionate intervention, is only beginning to experience a paradigm shift because middle-class, *white*, suburban children are showing up in seedy neighborhoods to cop heroin to avoid withdrawal, and not infrequently dying in the process. By virtue of the social phenomenon known as *proximity empathy*, black and brown lives have now *also* begun to matter, if only incidentally.

The greatest danger currently at the fore as the cresting wave of opioid addiction bears down upon us lies in the potential for us to fail to seize this moment where opportunity meets chance, and instead continue to have the wrong discussions, fail to make the necessary changes, and codify non-evidence based solutions that will serve to continue to upend not only the lives of the victims we seek to save, but of their families and of society as a whole. Society must resolve the Cartesian duality of mind vs. body and wholly reject the fundamentalist Christian attitude that human suffering of this variety is the result of sin, and in the minds of too many, that shunning of the sinner is approved by God. [20]

The acquisition of opioid addiction is very frequently due to an individual with a pre-disposition having had an excess of Adverse Childhood Experiences (ACEs), not to mention the far higher rates of mental illness in this population when compared with normal controls (see Appendix II). In addition, it is uncommon for individuals to become addicted iatrogenically (i.e., via their doctors Rx) after suffering a physical malady for which they were legitimately treated for pain with an opioid, especially when treated in an inpatient setting.

This itself is an entirely different situation from pain patients who are dependent on their pain medications because while this population, too, may suffer withdrawal symptoms upon discontinuation, there is clearly a much milder course of withdrawal for these patients, and most are tapered off of their pain medications without addiction ever becoming an issue. This fact alone would indicate that opioid addicted individuals are uniquely vulnerable to the aversive aspects of withdrawal, so much so that they will do anything to avoid it, while for dependent patients, withdrawal is experienced as something on the level of a bad cold or influenza.

The fact that these distinctions are lost upon physicians is a tragic confounding element that effectively means that most physicians are themselves prone to view opioid addiction in its current manifestation in the States as being almost 100% due to iatrogenic addiction, and thus to vastly over-estimate their individual contribution to the current epidemic of opioid addiction. This, in turn, has had a brutally chilling effect on physicians willingness to continue prescribing opioids for their chronic pain patients, most notably in light of the *disastrous* recommendations for opioid prescribing issued by the Centers for Disease Control in 2016 (see Appendix IV & Chapter 10).

While the core subject of this book is MMT, the current pain crisis in the U.S. must also be addressed as these are overlapping issues, and people would be well reminded to realize that one day it may be *them or their loved one* who requires intense pain relief. To leave the current group of neglected pain patients to their own devices is just as cruel as ruthlessly stigmatizing other humans. The sad irony is that many chronic pain patients are now seen, first and foremost, through the distorted glasses of drug-seeking behavior, and this appears to be essentially irrespective of how long they have been on opioid therapy or for actual cause. The harassment must stop. Now.

6

MYTHS ABOUT METHADONE
MAINTENANCE TREATMENT: THE
STIGMATIZATION OF A MEDICATION

To any objective observer, there is a large body of myths about and surrounding methadone. The tenacious persistence of these myths is difficult to understand let alone explain, however, some demographic factors may play a causal role in their development and persistence. We would like to preface this explanation with a caveat, and that is that even though we are discussing certain commonalities among opioid addicted individuals, the critical point that cannot be overlooked or underestimated is how contrary to stereotypes this highly heterogeneous population really is. In other words, while what is stated may apply to many opioid addicted individuals, by no means does this indicate that this applies to *all* of them. Opioid addiction is no stranger to any demographic.

As for the main body of those addicted to opioids, however, the following can *generally* be said: a large percentage of opioid addicted individuals come from a lower socioeconomic background than does your average citizen, although this has been changing due to the current opioid epidemic. To be more specific, they tend to lack in formal education, the importance of which can best be understood when looking at Piaget's stages of childhood mental development. Of the four stages, the salient point here is that the last stage, known as the formal operational stage is not attained by all adults, irrespective of whether they go on to develop an addiction or not. This skewing tends to be particularly strong in opioid addicted populations wherein the third of Piaget's stages, the concrete operation stage, is the last stage that they will have attained, therefore precluding more abstract thinking and the ability to abstract in general. This is not taught in school, this is developed in healthy homes with healthy primary caregivers. [50]

Compounding this disadvantage, a sizable percentage of these patients also lack anything beyond a primary education. The reasons for this demographic skewing amongst opioid addicted individuals is complex, but some commonalities are often in play, the most frequent one being that many opioid addicted individuals come from broken or highly dysfunctional families wherein, more often than not, poverty is the defining feature of their socioeconomic status.

This poverty can be considered to oftentimes encompass more than just a family's finances, such as dysfunctional primary relationships, communities with few if any resources in place to buttress the effects of poverty and neglect, and the fact that demographically similar family groups tend to aggregate just as other socioeconomic classes do, leaving vulnerable addicted individuals with a dearth of resources and, more often than not, surrounded by global dysfunction. When one is trying to survive this maelstrom of environmental insults, studying and homework rank low on the list of priorities. How can we, in good conscience, blame defenseless children (as adults) for their own arbitrary station in life?

"For the great enemy of truth is very often not the lie—deliberate, contrived, and dishonest—but the myth—persistent, persuasive, and unrealistic. Too often we hold fast to the clichés of our forebears. We subject all facts to a prefabricated set of interpretations. We enjoy the comfort of opinion without the discomfort of thought." John Kennedy, Yale University.

METHADONE IS A SUBSTITUTE FOR HEROIN
OR PRESCRIPTION OPIOIDS

Patients who are on a stable dose of methadone and who are not using any other non-prescribed or illicit medications are not addicted to the methadone. This is a logical fallacy, as addiction requires a loss of control over use and cravings for the drug, not to mention using despite adverse consequences, all of which do not occur when a patient is properly stabilized on methadone.

It is not an exaggeration to say that comparing the two is like comparing apples with footballs. People who take methadone as part of methadone maintenance treatment are *dependent* on it, not *addicted,* but this is the whole point of the treatment after all. One cannot glean the benefits of MMT without having to take methadone, but that's where the resemblance ends. [8]

After all, are not diabetics dependent on their daily insulin shots? What about hypertensives and their necessary dependence on their medication, not to mention psychiatric patients and their dependence on medication? How are these any different from being dependent on methadone?

METHADONE ROTS TEETH AND BONES

An equally persistent if not destructive myth is that methadone will rot ones teeth and bones. To say that this myth has no basis in fact is an understatement. The question as to how this myth arose can best be answered by a combination of two factors.

First, it is not uncommon in untreated opioid addicted individuals to see a marked decrease in personal hygiene, the teeth being no exception, and secondly, in many cases oral hygiene is the first aspect of personal hygiene to suffer. As such, by the time most people arrive at an MMT clinic, they are often already in some stage of periodontal disease or on the cusp of developing it. At worst, like all opioids, methadone may provide an aggravating factor to an already bad oral hygiene situation by causing a side effect known as xerostomia, also known as dry mouth. Considering this, a certain amount of saliva is necessary in order to maintain adequate oral hygiene, and saliva, as such, acts as a protective barrier between tooth enamel and bacteria.

That being said, it is a long way off from having a case of dry mouth to obtaining a mouth full of rotting teeth. In the vast majority of individuals stabilized on MMT, simply practicing good oral hygiene and keeping ones mouth well-moistened with over the counter products such as Biotene will render one no more likely to develop dental disease than anyone else in the general population.

As to the origin of the "bone rotting" myth, there is a high index of suspicion that some people interpret the musculoskeletal pain that is experienced upon withdrawal from opioids, including methadone, as some form of permanent damage to their bones, when in fact such pain does not originate from the bones and will pass with the conclusion of the withdrawal phenomenon itself. The pain interpreted as bone pain is actually generalized musculoskeletal pain that arises because during withdrawal, one does not have a fully functioning endorphin system to take care of everyday aches and pains. It is the long term use of opioids that causes this metabolic disturbance, because the brain is receiving hormonal messages from the outside world telling it that it need no longer needs to produce its own endogenous morphine, a.k.a., endorphins. Without this endogenous production, the withdrawal or underdosing of methadone will leave one feeling achy and generally miserable because one no longer possess an intact internal pain relief system. All relief essentially is exogenous in this population in the form of the opioid, be it methadone or any other opioid.

METHADONE WAS NAMED IN "HONOR" OF ADOLF HITLER...
One of the truly bizarre and paranoid myths surrounding methadone is that it was named after Adolf Hitler. Surprisingly, rumblings about this myth can not infrequently be heard among addicted individuals and even members of the treatment community. The origin of this myth is rooted in a linguistic misunderstanding. When methadone was first commercially produced one of the first proprietary names was Dolophine, which is Latin for, "an end to pain." Where people were clearly misled was in believing the fabricated story that the name Dolophine itself was named to honor A*dolph* Hitler, which of course has a vague plausibility in that methadone was invented during WWII in Germany, but that's where the myth meets the end of the road.

METHADONE MAKES MEN STERILE
This is an unfortunate and serious myth, most particularly prevalent within the African American community, regarding the physical effects of methadone and the long term consequences of its administration on gamete

formation. It is understandable that this community, particularly after the Tuskegee Syphilis Experiment, is less than fully trusting of large governmental institutions, particularly medical bodies that are entrusted with their care. The problem for the dawning of the 21ˢᵗ century and those caught up in the attendant opioid epidemic is that myths like this are persistent, difficult to correct and deadly in their impact.

To add to the unfortunate confusion is the fact that methadone, when taken long-term, can indeed have physical side-effects, like every opioid does, one of which is the *potential* suppression of the hypothalamic-pituitary-gonadal axis. The result of this suppression can lead to a decrease in the amount of sex hormones produced in the body. Testosterone levels produced in both men and women *can* dwindle and can lead to a corresponding decrease in both sex drive and sperm production. For women, estrogen production may also suffer, which can first lead to a disturbance in the normal menstrual cycle, and later, the eventual development of amenorrhea, or the absence of a menstrual cycle. These effects are reversible after a period of withdrawal.

We must differentiate among the opioids, however, because this kind of endocrine instability is seen as a rule in addicted individuals that have an opioid habit that they are sustaining through the use of short acting, full mu-agonists like heroin, morphine, Dilaudid, fentanyl, etc. One could almost call the phenomenon consumers undergo an opioid-induced "endocrine roller coaster," because about three times a day, what an individual who is active in their addiction does is send an abort signal to the part of their brain that is responsible for the modulation of the most crucial intuitive drives and the maintenance of the most essential procreative and survival instruments by turning the hormone production switch off.

Ultimately, all opioids can disturb the brain's ability to maintain equilibrium or homeostasis. All other things being equal, however, it must be emphasized that with long-term or indefinite maintenance treatment with methadone, though the effect on the endocrine system is similar, its impact remains the most negligible when compared to other full mu-opioids like those previously mentioned. (e.g. heroin, morphine, hydromorphone, fentanyl, etc.). This is due to methadone's extremely unique pharmacology, which though potentially disruptive to the equilibrium of the gonadotrophic hormones, is the least so in its class. This may be of small comfort to the opioid user, to be sure, however, he must regularly be assessed and reminded that what he is experiencing is normal, expected, and directly related to the fact that he is taking an opioid period. It comes with the territory.

A decrease in libido is neither absolute nor definite. Once again, this is where individual differences in physiology, as well as psychological factors, come heavily into play. A loss of interest in sex can be a difficult challenge for some methadone patients to overcome, particularly for those in committed relationships or in relationships where both partners are in a maintenance program, but it is possible to manage with alternative therapies that involve Testosterone supplementation and Erectile Dysfunction medications. Considering that the alternative is being six feet under or in a six foot cell, the tradeoff for the decrease in sex drive is more than worth it.

Being in MMT precludes one from driving a car or operating heavy machinery/Patients who are stable on their methadone dose, who are not using other non-prescribed or illicit drugs, are not able to perform well in many jobs.

This particular myth is somewhat easier to understand superficially since the fundamental underlying assumption regarding methadone is that it is a psychoactive drug, and thus were one to take it, one would become sufficiently impaired to preclude one from undertaking any potentially dangerous activities like driving.

In the most literal sense, this assumption does hold true, meaning that for a neophyte or someone who has no tolerance to opioids, the consumption of methadone would result in discernible intoxication, and the attendant warnings against operating a car or heavy machinery would be warranted.

The patient in an MMT clinic presents an entirely different picture, however. For most, the patient will enter the clinic with a tolerance to opioids, then as the proper protocol is followed and the dosage increased, the patient will soon develop a complete tolerance to any of the psychoactive effects of methadone, so much so that it would be impossible for an objective observer to detect and for the patient himself to perceive. For this individual, methadone will become no different from a daily multivitamin in its psychoactive potential.

METHADONE MAINTENANCE PATIENTS ARE "LOSERS"

Another pervasive and especially corrosive myth is that individuals who participate in MMT programs are society's losers. Unfortunately, this seems to be almost the default assumption among far too many neurotypicals and even among some addicted individuals themselves.

The origins of this myth are as simple to explain as they are to dispel. They lie in a phenomenon known in psychology as *confirmation bias*. Like the phrase implies, the affected individual has a bias wherein they only see evidence that confirms their preexisting belief, thus when confronted with evidence that challenges that belief, they simply dismiss it out of hand since it doesn't confirm their preexisting bias or notion.

Examples of this abound in everyday life, for instance, when was the last time that you saw a "feel good" news story about a successful MMT patient? Of course the answer is most likely *never once*, since stories like that don't sell papers or play to an audience that is hungry for salacious and "juicy," extreme news stories. After eight years of concerted research, the author found exactly _one_ newspaper article that spoke unequivocally of the many success stories, and it was published in 1999... [45]

People will constantly be exposed, however, to negative images of opioid addicted individuals and MMT patients, because their failures fit the dominant narrative perfectly, and thus further serve to confirm an already existing bias. The reality is that patients stably maintained on methadone for long periods of time can be found in essentially all walks of life. Unfortunately we will never hear about their stories and their successes precisely because they are so guarded against revealing their status as an MMT patient given the existing stigma, stereotypes, and discrimination.

The very thought of revealing ones MMT status is so powerfully aversive that to date, *not one single person of note* has come forward with the admission that they are a current MMT patient. That this is because none exist strains credulity, given the very high rates of substance use and abuse in the entertainment industry alone. It is one of society's last remaining scarlet letters which no one wishes to wear.

PREGNANT WOMEN SHOULD NOT TAKE METHADONE/ METHADONE IS NOT ADVISABLE FOR PREGNANT WOMEN

The tragic irony of this myth is that, in point of fact, the exact *opposite* is true and it does not require much reflection to see why. First of all, an untreated opioid addicted woman who is pregnant is already using opioids, and that use of opioids frequently involves intravenous injections. As to how someone could think it would be better to leave a pregnant woman to her own devices or to the sheer force of her willpower to stop using because she is with child is a mystery, since the fact of the matter is that she will continue to use opioids, and thus what will also continue to occur is that the developing fetus will alternately be exposed to a cycle of intoxication followed by withdrawal, and may quite possibly become infected with a transmissible disease.

Withdrawal during pregnancy can be harmful to the fetus and can even result in spontaneous abortion, as the body's entire endocrine system is violently out of whack due to the impact that short acting opioids can have on it. It is well known that opioids can suppress the hypothalamic-pituitary-gonadal axis, whose homeostasis is crucial for maintaining a healthy pregnancy. If we contrast this chaos of the endocrine system on short acting opioids with the endocrine stabilization that is achieved on MMT, the choice for expecting mothers should be self-evident.

The persistence of this myth is hard to understand, considering the risks to the unborn fetus of maternal heroin (or other opioid) use: HIV infection, fetal withdrawal syndrome, and sudden fetal death, among other equally unacceptable outcomes. The reality is that fetal survival and thriving are dependent upon the mother remaining abstinent from all illicit opioid use, and this is by far most easily and safely accomplished by placing the pregnant mother on a stabilizing dose of methadone. After the birth of the child, the baby can be weaned from the methadone using any one of a number of different weaning protocols. For those who have concerns that the baby will be born addicted to opioids, this must be immediately dispelled as babies, by definition, do not have the cognitive facility to even become addicted. Rather, when babies are born to mothers on methadone maintenance, they will display signs and symptoms of opioid *dependence* and as such can be weaned off the medication using shorter acting opioids like morphine, for pediatric metabolic reasons, until they are entirely opioid free. That this process may be mildly uncomfortable for the baby must be weighed against the very real risks that the baby is protected from, which includes the transmission of diseases such as HIV, Hepatitis C, Hepatitis B, etc., and potential birth defects.

METHADONE IS HARDER TO "KICK"

This particular myth is somewhat rooted in the reality of methadone's unique pharmacology. Since methadone persists in the body for a much longer period of time than do short acting opioids like heroin, morphine, Dilaudid, fentanyl, etc., the withdrawal process can take substantially longer to set in as well as to subside, however, the withdrawal process is accordingly less intense than it is with the shorter-acting opioids.

Stated somewhat differently, it takes longer to withdraw from methadone than it does from short-acting opioids. Some people prefer to "get it over with" in a "quick boil," while others prefer "kicking" on a "slow simmer." Either way, in both contexts, we're referring to people becoming abstinent via the cold-turkey route, something that is *never* to be recommended especially if the individual has a chronic health condition or is also on other medications like benzodiazepines. In these situations, cold-turkey withdrawal can prove fatal. [51, 52]

If one must withdraw from methadone, it is imperative to do so in under a doctor's supervision who can offer tapered doses over longer periods of time, but also bear in mind that the whole original point of MMT is that one remain on methadone *indefinitely*, since there are likely permanent metabolic changes to the brain in the addicted individual. The most benefit, by far, is to be had by indefinite MMT, but each person must decide in consultation with their treating physician what course of action is best for them. [42]

Methadone is "liquid handcuffs"

This particular myth is nonsensical, since having any kind of habit can be seen as a form of unwanted dependence, most particularly a heroin habit. So why the fuss over the legally created dependence of MMT? Our suspicion is that this has mostly to do with the thicket of federally stipulated rules and regulations which can make a person's first 90-180 days in particular very difficult, especially if they already have regular employment.

The difficulties one may encounter in continuing one's employment during the first 90-180 days of MMT are very real, and this must be acknowledged in a newer, updated version of the federal regulations. The stress on employed individuals first starting MMT can be overwhelming, and this needs to be addressed for the future if MMT is to be made more widely available (see Appendix I).

Severe consequences are what will
Really keep people from relapsing

What is baffling about this particular myth is its sheer persistence, despite all evidence to the contrary. Belief in this appears to be particularly widespread within certain sub-sectors of law-enforcement and the religious community. The reality is that no amount of aversive consequences will keep an opioid addicted individual abstinent "for good." To best illustrate this, I will quote Dr. Gabor Mate, a cutting-edge addiction specialist, addressing the sheer futility of imposing "consequences".

'...we have built a system that thinks we will stop addicts by *increasing* their pain. "If I had to design a system that was intended to keep people addicted, I'd design exactly the system we have right now," Gabor would tell me. "I'd attack people, and ostracize them." He has seen that "the more you stress people, the more they're going to use. The more you de-stress people, the less they're going to use. So to create a system where you ostracize and marginalize and criminalize people, and force them to live in poverty with disease, you are basically guaranteeing that they will stay at it."

"If negative consequences led people to transformation then I wouldn't have a single patient left," he says, "because they've experienced every negative consequence in the book. Being jailed. Being beaten up. Being traumatized.

Being hurt. HIV. Hepatitis C. Poverty." Gabor looks at me, his eyes sagging a little, as if picturing it all, "What *haven't* they suffered yet?" [23]

METHADONE CLINICS ARE JUST A SOURCE OF DIVERSION FOR METHADONE

This myth unfortunately feeds off of the stereotype of the opioid addicted individual as a craven, amoral sub-human who will do anything for heroin. What makes this myth so very unfortunate is that it is absolutely not reflected in the statistics.

In point of fact, almost all deaths attributable to methadone have been due exclusively to the pill form which can be prescribed for pain by any doctor and obtained at any pharmacy. The lack of methadone provided by clinics that is diverted for purchase on the street is partially a function of the fact that it is just not nearly as sought after as other drugs. For whatever reason, oral methadone is tough to abuse and therefore not a serious target for the black market.

As for diversion from within the clinic, this is nearly impossible as the DEA regularly and randomly audits clinic prescribing records down to the very milligram, with every drop needing to be accounted for. To top this off, federal regulations require that the methadone be stored in massive, bank-like vault safes so burglary is out of the question. As it now stands, methadone clinics don't attract crime, they prevent it.

METHADONE PATIENTS DON'T REQUIRE PAIN MEDICATIONS

This myth used to be much more prevalent *in the general medical community* because of a poor understanding of how opioid analgesia in general, and methadone analgesia specifically, are slightly different if somewhat overlapping.

It used to be that the general consensus was, particularly among primary care physicians, that because methadone prevents withdrawal and cravings for at least 24 hours, it must also have an equivalently long-acting analgesic effect. This is, in point of fact, not true. In a methadone stabilized patient, they may derive analgesic benefit for about six hours after dosing, but no more as after that the analgesic effect wears off.

This is why it's crucial for medical personnel to administer short-acting opioids like morphine or hydromorphone to MMT patients if they are hospitalized and in pain, as their daily methadone dose will not provide the effective analgesia necessary for good, rapid healing. Two caveats apply here; first, the dose of short-acting opioid must be larger than that for someone with no tolerance and secondly, the short-acting opioid must usually be administered at slightly shorter intervals than it would be for someone with no tolerance as tolerance to methadone both diminishes the short acting opioid's peak effect as well as their duration of action.

There is absolutely no excuse not to give opioid analgesics to MMT patients in severe pain. After all, fear of creating an addiction is an entirely moot point, so withholding analgesia in this context is nothing less than cruel when severe pain is present.

THE METHADONE PATIENT WILL REQUIRE EVER-INCREASING DOSES TO SATISFY THEIR CRAVINGS

This myth is absurd precisely because there is currently a problem with MMT patients requesting that their doses be *lowered*, not increased, and this can lead to the danger of relapse. It is rare to hear an MMT patient say, "My dose is not enough," so fixated are so many of them on reducing their doses, sometimes with good reason, sometimes not. Even though they are given a certain degree of flexibility over their daily methadone dose, it is extremely rare to hear of patients wanting to increase it indefinitely. It just doesn't happen in real-world MMT clinics.

In reality, even opioid addicts with unlimited access to heroin eventually stabilize on a given dose of heroin, and even decrease their total daily dose. [23]

THE BOTTOM LINE, TAKE-AWAY MESSAGE FROM THE NATIONAL INSTITUTES OF HEALTH (N.I.H.)

To drive home a critical point which raises as many questions as it answers, the following *consensus statement* by the N.I.H., no less, *published in 1997*, a statement issued by a conference of veritable experts on opioid addiction, is testimony to how very long the truth about the nature of opioid addiction, and its effective treatment with indefinite MMT, has really been quietly known throughout the academic medical world. Though even this star panel had difficulty staying on track with respect to the correct terminology ("dependence" when they mean addiction, etc.), their ultimate message was loud and clear.

"Once dependence (*sic*) is established, there are usually repeated cycles of cessation and relapse extending over decades. This "addiction career" is often accompanied by periods of imprisonment....*Although a drug-free state represents an optimal treatment goal, research has demonstrated that this goal <u>cannot be achieved or sustained by the majority of opiate-dependent people</u>. However, other laudable treatment goals, including decreased drug use, reduced criminal activity, and gainful employment can be achieved by most MMT patients.*...The most striking evidence of the positive impact of MMT on death rates is studies directly comparing these rates in opiate-dependent persons, on and off methadone. *Every study* showed that death rates were lower in opiate-dependent persons maintained on methadone compared with those who were not. The median death rate for opiate-dependent persons in MMT was 30 percent of the death rate of those not in treatment. *A clear consequence of <u>not</u> treating opiate dependence, therefore, is a death rate that is more than three times greater than that experienced by those engaged in MMT.*" [135] (ed. note: *emphasis added*)

7

ELIMINATION OF
DOSAGE CEILINGS

Dosage ceilings are, as the name implies, upper and arbitrary limits on the daily dose which a methadone patient can take that are established by clinic owners. This problem has certainly not been helped by the fact that methadone treatment is operated entirely outside the realm of normal medical practice (see Appendix I, §8.12, sub. a-f, Title 42 Code of Federal Regulations), and as such, exists in a kind of vacuum of medical information. Though the information on proper dosing protocol is widely available, each clinician must seek it out for themselves. If there is any confirmation bias at play, the likelihood of that clinician searching for more information on dosing is diminishingly small.

The result this vacuum produces is the sincere, if entirely false belief on the part of some clinicians that a certain number of milligrams should be "more than enough" methadone to treat any opioid addicted individual. The reality, of course, is much more complex and does not, in fact, subscribe to this particular school of thought. As a result, if you are a patient who is unfortunate enough to find oneself at a clinic which imposes dosage ceilings, and if you happen to be a patient known to be a "rapid metabolizer," then a successful outcome on MMT may be impossible to achieve. [22,28]

A rapid metabolizer on an insufficient dose of methadone can expect to experience withdrawal symptoms before their next dose is due, which can sometimes occur many hours beforehand. This raises the issue of a relapse hazard, of using again to alleviate withdrawal symptoms. This, of course, suggests that the user may resort to obtaining an opioid from illicit channels, which makes the entire point of the maintenance program moot.

What is a rapid metabolizer? A rapid metabolizer is a person for whom a more typical methadone dosage simply does not suffice to control their withdrawal symptoms and cravings for a full 24 hours, the reason being that for genetically predetermined factors entirely outside of the addicted individuals control, their livers metabolize methadone much more rapidly than the more average opioid addicted individual's liver.

What this means as it concerns methadone is that the liver works overtime to eliminate it from the body, and there is no way around this accelerated function outside of an upward adjustment in the dose of methadone administered. The range of methadone doses in normal individuals should help to make it clear that one size cannot and does not fit all. There *are* patients who can be maintained on 60 milligrams or less of methadone a day indefinitely. These patients, however, are statistically in the minority, similar to how rapid metabolizers also make up only a minority of the total MMT population. Statistically speaking, the distribution of adequate doses in any large enough sample of an MMT population tends to follow what is known as a normal distribution, colloquially speaking, a "bell curve." [22]

The more average maintenance dose tends to be around 100 to 150 milligrams, depending upon the individual MMT clinic's dosing policies, however it is not unusual in more enlightened clinics who treat rapid metabolizers to administer maintenance doses, albeit rarely, upwards of 400 milligrams a day. [28] It should be made clear that clinicians will know when they've achieved *approximately* the correct dose when they analyze blood serum levels. For example, if at 8:00 a.m. 400 mg is administered to Patient A and 80 mg is administered to Patient B, they could very well have *identical* blood plasma levels four hours later, controlling for all other factors. Individuals can differ in their abilities to clear methadone from their bodies by a factor of *100-fold*. [22,31]

That having been said, serum methadone levels (SML) have their limitations. They are not necessarily *always* reflective of an adequate dose, even if the results come back in the therapeutic range, so it still is critical for the underdosed patient to be given wide latitude in the determination of what a "holding dose" is for them. That this places the patient in an adversarial position ("It's your word against these 'objective' serum levels'") can be difficult to get past and is part of the unfortunate reality that bedevils this issue. Patients should ultimately be taken at their word, especially when they display some more objective signs of withdrawal such as dilated pupils, a runny nose, watery eyes, tremors, etc. [22,28,34,31]

As an example, it is commonly believed that a serum methadone level (SML) is the objective way to ascertain if someone's dose is enough, and that in this respect, the "numbers don't lie." While it is true that numbers don't lie, one has to ask what, exactly, are those numbers telling us?

For reasons beyond the scope of this book, any given dose of methadone is really made up of two types of molecules, in a 50:50 ratio. These two molecules are identical except for the fact that they are mirror-images of one another (think of a right and left hand, how they're the same, yet different.)

In the real-world, only one of the mirror-images produces all of the opioid effects commonly associated with methadone, and it is the left-handed form. The problem this creates for blood SML tests is that the test cannot distinguish between the active and inactive forms of methadone: It simply reflects the sum total of *both* molecules, even though it is known that they are metabolized or broken down *at differing rates in different people*, and that the right-handed molecule is inactive as an opioid. [22]

"Given that as many as 30–40% of Caucasian and African populations carry at least one rs3745274 minor allele and the confounding nature of this genotype on "total" methadone levels, *this calls to question whether therapeutic drug monitoring using a non-stereoselective assay could be meaningfully interpreted.*" [34] [ed. note: *emphases added*]

"Moreover, as Table 2 demonstrates, there was no apparent correlation between methadone dose and SML." [22,31]

What this effectively means in the context of an SML is that the clinician is not getting nearly the precise information he needs from this measurement. This is why it is so important when titrating to a correct dose to go by SML's *in addition to* subjective clinical signs and symptoms. To judge a dose by SML alone is very hit-or-miss, again, depending upon the patient's individual metabolism. [22]

This is the current reality of methadone maintenance treatment and it is also arguably the biggest factor at play as to why some patients will "fail" at clinics that rely solely on the blood SML to determine appropriate dosing caps. It is simply because they are literally not receiving the therapeutic benefits of methadone and are therefore effectively *not even really being treated.* This leaves these patients and their families with the notion that methadone maintenance doesn't work or that they are personal failures, while also leaving their treatment providers with the erroneous notion that the patient is not committed to their own recovery when nothing could be further from the truth. One shudders to think of how many addicted individuals have had to die simply because of these arbitrary dosage ceilings, and how many patients and families have been destroyed. [30,33]

What is particularly unfortunate about dosage ceilings and the havoc that they can wreak on people's lives is that there are plenty of studies from academia showing *vastly* better outcomes at clinics where dosage ceilings are not codified, and yet there are still far too many clinicians out there who firmly *believe* low dosages to be effective. [33,53]

We can lead a horse to water, but we seemingly have not succeeded in leading physicians to continuing medical education. At this point in time, the general consensus appears to be that the medical establishment has failed in this regard.

Ironically, there do exist studies that show no benefit between "high dose" versus "low dose" MMT. However, upon closer inspection it must be noted that what are defined as high doses in these studies are 100 mg daily doses. This was the very *lowest* dose used by Dole and Nyswander for maintenance, and so it should come as little surprise that with the dosing bar set so low, outcomes will continue to *tend* to be poorer when there are upper limits imposed upon patients as to a daily dosage when that dosage is pre-determined rather than individualized. [28,29,30,42]

"The Effects of Dosage on Methadone Maintenance Treatment— Research regarding methadone dosage levels clearly establishes that low average doses are inappropriate in methadone maintenance treatment. No single level is effective for all patients, although NIDA-supported research has suggested that the minimum effective dosage for most methadone maintenance patients is 60 mg per day. The specific dosage for a patient cannot be determined arbitrarily because patients metabolize methadone at different rates. In addition, the appropriate dosage can change over time or in response to specific situations such as pregnancy or the use of other medications. Overall, methadone dosage should be based on the patient's individual needs, goals of treatment, and progress in treatment.

In the Ball and Ross studies (1991), illicit opioid use was directly related to methadone dosage levels."

"Methadone dose should not be rapidly increased or decreased—or used in contingency management—because such changes tend to disrupt the normalization of physiological function achieved by steady dose treatment. *If the stabilized methadone dose/plasma levels are disrupted, drug hunger and drug-seeking behaviors are likely to reappear.*" [29] [ed. note: *emphasis added*]

The very real need to follow the original Dole-Nyswander protocols of MMT clashes with the current reality of each methadone clinic as an island unto itself. Why some clinicians think that they can achieve better results than the very people who developed the protocol with such efficacious results, namely, Dr.s Vincent Dole and Marie Nyswander, is difficult to comprehend let alone blindly accept.

Shockingly, a 1988 survey of U.S. methadone clinics found that 70% of them maintained patients at doses of *50 mg/day or less*. Ten years later, in 1998, the average dose was 69.4 mg/day. These are troubling statistics, but they go a long way toward explaining why MMT in the U.S. is not producing the consistently good outcomes that we know are possible when dosage ceilings are not implemented. As can be seen from the numbers, under-dosing is a vast problem in a large number of U.S. MMT facilities. [28,29,54,55]

The naturalistic question at this point is, "what should a patient who happens to be a rapid metabolizer do when confronted with this ceiling?"

One answer currently available as a solution is to leave that clinic for one that does not impose dosage ceilings. This is, however, far easier said than done because as it currently stands, there are a limited number of these facilities in the States, and as such, only patients who have the means to endure long commutes can avail themselves of their services. In fact, for a distressing number of patients seeking to avail themselves of this treatment modality, they must commute multiple hours to and from these clinics.

Furthermore, since many patients are unaware of what the actual protocols are for good, effective MMT, they oftentimes indirectly assist a clinic in improperly treating them because they cannot effectively advocate on their own behalf. One of the most common issues that can be heard among people talking about at methadone clinics is their dosage level, specifically how they think it is too high and how they want to "taper-off" of the methadone. This dichotomy between what is and what should ideally be must be bridged with information and the destigmatization of "high" dosage numbers.

Effective methadone maintenance depends upon a few factors, arguably the most salient being proper dosage, and in this situation, more is very often precisely what is needed instead of less. To anyone wondering why, the answer is straightforward; when MMT was developed, the whole idea was to create enough tolerance in the addicted individual so that additional opioids have no rewarding effect, then give a large enough dose to block cravings and finally to eliminate the physical need for opioids so that day-to-day functional living can occur. When Dole and Nyswander worked on the original methadone maintenance experiment, the average daily dose was 100-150 mg. Nowadays it is not uncommon to see people on 80 or even 60 mg doses, which are generally not enough for both full opioid "blockade" and craving control. That these patients often end-up as treatment "failures" should not surprise any health professional. [28,29,42,56]

In all fairness, it must be mentioned that just as there are ultra-rapid metabolizers, there are also ultra-slow metabolizers, and it is for this small sub-group that a dosage of between 40-80 mg is absolutely effective. That being said, most MMT patients fall somewhere in the middle of the normal statistical distribution, meaning that most patients will do well on dosages between 90-150 mg, approximately speaking. [29]

One important point that can't be overlooked is that the problems with dosage ceilings arise only *because* MMT methadone is ingested orally. Without getting too complicated, oral ingestion of any medication will bring about what is known as a "first-pass effect" by the liver, before it ever gets into someone's bloodstream. What this effectively means is that with some medications, this first-pass effect can remove up to 90+% of the ingested medication from the body before it ever enters a persons circulation, the degree to which the drug is metabolized being mostly determined by the chemical nature of the medication and, to a lesser extent, the genetic variability of the metabolizing enzymes in each person's liver. For example, with heroin or morphine, this first-pass effect removes about 70% of the orally ingested dose before it ever hits the bloodstream, which is one of the main reasons why this route of administration is never used with illicit opioids. It's simply too wasteful for such expensive drugs. [22]

With methadone, it is a general rule of thumb that 50% of an orally ingested dose is lost to first-pass metabolism, which simply means that in order to achieve the effects of 100 mg of oral methadone, one would require only about 50 mg by injection. For this reason, a given dose of heroin given by injection or snorting, which both circumvent first pass metabolism, can have equivalent effects on a vastly heterogeneous group of consumers. Not so with orally administered methadone. [22] This is by no means an argument for allowing methadone to be administered by injection, as the entire idea of MMT is to move an at risk person away from risky behaviors like intravenous drug injection. It is simply another explanation for why dosage ceilings are cruel and arbitrary.

The good news is that in 2005 the federal regulations were updated to expressly forbid what they refer to as "dosage caps," but the bad news is that enforcement of this particular regulation appears to be particularly lax. [30] Why there would be such a non-binding attitude among regulators over such a life-and-death issue is a mystery, but that is the current situation.

Rapid metabolizers have one option left before having to resort to utilizing creative measures and this option is something known as split-dosing. As the name implies, a given daily dose is split into two doses taken separately during the day. The only underlying assumption with respect to utilizing this technique is that one is already receiving a reasonable sized dose of *at least* 100 mg. This number really is a minimum for successful split-dosing, when it works. While this method of administration can and does work for some people, for others it does nothing to resolve the early "breakthrough withdrawal." So much is dependent on individual physiology that one-size-fits-all recommendations cannot be made with respect to this issue. [22,29]

If one does happen to be a rapid metabolizer, perhaps the consolation here is that one does have federal regulations on ones side, so that if enough waves are made, arriving at a correct maintenance dose is possible. It may, however, require one to submit to a series of peak and trough blood levels drawn for every 10 mg increase in dose, something which will both have to be done at personal cost and which can take a good chunk of time, at least until one reaches their effective dose.

One final point: if you happen to live in the state of Tennessee, you might as well go straight to the State Opioid Treatment Authority (SOTA) to make your case, if you are a rapid metabolizer, since this is the only state in the union to have codified a dosage cap of 120 mg in their state regulations. [57] It's not clear at this point if this is a direct violation of federal law, though one would surmise that it is given the guidelines issued in 2012. It may require a case to go through the district courts in order to challenge this contravention.

8

PROBLEMS WITH
METHADONE MAINTENANCE
TREATMENT DELIVERY

Even though there is a highly regulated and official delivery system for methadone within the context of maintenance treatment, it is, unfortunately, a system that is quite broken and in need of repair. To understand how methadone maintenance treatment is broken in the U.S., it would help to look at how it began and consider the conditions under which it was created.

The year was 1970 when then-President Richard Nixon had declared a full-on war on drugs, and he enlisted the help of health professionals in doing so. Thus, the MMT which had still been experimental in 1966 became officially legislated into law in the U.S. with the passage of the Drug Abuse Prevention Office and Treatment Act of 1972 (Public Law 92-255, March 21, 1972). Crucial to bear in mind is that the statutes are federal and as such, states do not have any options regarding their enforcement *with the exception that they can be more severe* in their implementation than the federal laws actually dictate.

These federal statutes, while containing a fundamental element of fairness within them, nonetheless show clear marks of having been written during a time which was reactionary. In light of this, many of the rules clearly reflect attitudes and feelings which were, at the time, running extremely high, and they display a certain measure of "better to be too strict than not strict enough." (see Appendix 1) Most salient to this book are the practical implications of this legislation's effect on the lives of everyday ordinary Americans who require MMT.

One issue which has been overlooked by legislators is the very real issue of payment for MMT services. Just like the rest of the U.S. healthcare system, payment must somehow be arranged between a patient and one's clinic before treatment can commence. Fortunately and at least for now, a number of states have Medicaid "block grants" which are used to fund private and non-profit MMT clinics, meaning that patients pay about $20 a week for services rendered, but if one happens to live in a state without such a grant in operation, or if one doesn't qualify for such grant monies, one may have to pay entirely out-of-pocket. The average private cost per week of methadone treatment is between $60-$80, which is not an insubstantial amount of money for most opioid addicted individuals.

The unfortunate reality is that precisely during this time of the opioid epidemic, legislators are not putting money where it is needed. Instead, they are essentially throwing pennies at the problem, and this translates directly into less MMT treatment availability for those who need it most. This is a disturbing state of affairs whose trend line doesn't have a positive trajectory. [58,59]

Cost will be the first obstacle one will have to overcome upon entering a methadone maintenance treatment program, but it should not be prohibitive to an individuals admission. As there is little to nothing patients can do to avoid costs one way or the other, it is suggested that, if necessary, the new MMT patient start a budget which factors in the cost of their treatment. This may be very difficult for some people, but in the U.S. it is currently the only solution towards this issue. Until universal healthcare-as-a-human-right for all is codified, treatment cost will be a sticking point for a number of patients.

Perhaps the single largest factor that all U.S. MMT programs share in common is that they are each run entirely separately and *outside of the regular healthcare delivery system*. This was intentional and by design, considering the stigmatization of addicted individuals at the time the program was established. An unintended consequence of this is that while there is federal oversight of each clinic, it is by far mostly oversight that is directed towards ensuring that no diversion of methadone take place, and as such consists of regular visits by the DEA to go over inventory, stock, records, etc. (see Appendix I)

The same cannot be said for oversight of the therapeutic activities of the individual MMT clinic. This has led to the current reality that each clinic is really a separate autonomous unit unto itself in that, while there are certain commonalities dictated by federal law regarding the dispensing of methadone, all other therapeutic activities are almost entirely developed and administered at the discretion of the individual clinic, the net result of this being that even clinics in the same town can have vastly different treatment philosophies and, accordingly, vastly different outcomes for patients. (see Chapter 16)

There are essentially two differing clinic "philosophies," and which one an individual attempting to address his opioid addiction can end up with is more often than not due to the luck of the draw. This is why doing ones homework regarding potential clinics can be so important. One doesn't want to end up at a clinic where the philosophy is to stabilize a patient for a given period of time with the eventual goal of tapering them to abstinence, if ones goal is instead long-term, indefinite maintenance. Ultimately, if one is lucky, the choice will be up to them, and it is suggested that one choose long-term MMT. People who taper to abstinence run an incredibly high risk of relapsing at some future point in time, and initial relapse is strongly correlated with risk for overdose. This is the experience of over 100 years of trying to keep opioid addicts abstinent. [20]

As another example of differences among clinics and providers, methadone Clinic A may require that patients perform urine drops every time that they dose to assess for any illicit drug use, whereas Clinic B may be satisfied with less frequent and more random urine testing – possibly even not testing for substances such as marijuana (the federal minimum is for testing only 8 times per calendar year). Marijuana is an excellent example of the tremendous confusion that reigns between Clinic A and Clinic B. For while it is "allowed" in Clinic A, in Clinic B, it is so strictly prohibited that one can have ones take-home privileges rescinded for testing positive, even if that state has legislated that it is permissible for medicinal use.

It might be worth remembering in this context that this is a situation where the federal statutes, as written, provide no relief because the states have the prerogative to implement *stricter* rules regarding methadone than the federal rules mandate e.g., Tennessee and Michigan are both more stringent than federal regulations stipulate. States are simply prohibited from making them *less onerous*.

At this point some readers may be wondering why even bother mentioning marijuana as an issue in MMT. As alluded to before, the reason is because in the past two decades mainstream medicine has come to embrace Cannabis as a legitimate treatment for a number of conditions, such as epilepsy, Crohn's disease, PTSD, and chronic, unremitting pain, among other diseases.

While this embrace has been somewhat tentative and regional, it has still been influential enough that a number of states have legalized marijuana for medical uses, and other states have gone so far as to legalize the use of marijuana for recreational purposes. For Clinic B, which happens to reside in such a medical marijuana state, one would wonder why they would even bother testing for marijuana if that patient has a valid condition and a doctor's prescription for its use?

The sad reality is that many MMT patients have some serious physical and/or psychiatric co-morbidities, and to cut them off from a treatment modality like medical Cannabis is ethically questionable, especially in light of the fact that in the U.S. many pharmaceutical medications to treat the aforementioned conditions are prohibitively expensive for precisely this population.

This brings us to the current legal oxymoron that marijuana happens to find itself in, for on a federal level, THC, the active ingredient in marijuana, falls under *two* different regulatory statutes depending only upon whether it is pharmaceutical THC or whether it is natural THC, the former being scheduled in Schedule III of the DEA's list of controlled substances, while the latter plant-based THC is still listed as a Schedule I controlled substance which, like heroin, LSD and mescaline, classifies it as a drug with *no acceptable medical use*.

The regulatory hypocrisy is both stunning and harmful. The reality for a patient who has to go to Clinic B essentially entails that even if they need marijuana medically, they cannot take it. Of course, the natural question arises as to why, if at this point it is legal on the state level, medical marijuana would even be prohibited at Clinic B. This is where the individuation of clinics comes into play.

The owner of Clinic A, while being perfectly aware of the aforementioned statutes, does not fear any repercussions from the DEA were he to allow some patients to take marijuana.

Contrast that with owner of Clinic B, who is so afraid of the repercussions from the DEA for letting a patient take marijuana, even though it is federally considered a Schedule III drug for certain patients, that he simply chooses to opt out of allowing *any* marijuana whatsoever to be used by his patients. This renders his patients vulnerable to the vicissitudes of their own diseases which they are trying to treat and accordingly increases, at the very least, their morbidity. Again, a revision of the federal regulations is what is clearly required if this problem is to be solved on a national basis.

An obvious solution to the marijuana problem is for the FDA and the DEA to finally reschedule marijuana into Schedule III and remove it from Schedule I status, as it shares literally no qualities with any of the other substances listed under Schedule I. This is easier said than done, however, as in years past we have seen a number of cases brought before federal courts seeking precisely such a change in scheduling status *fail*.

Up and until this writing, marijuana re-scheduling has not occurred both because legislators with neither a medical background nor expertise have exerted undue influence on the legislative process and are also subject to pressure exerted by organizations like Partnership for a Drug Free America, DARE, and certain religious groups. Until we can disentangle the medical aspect from the "moral" aspect of marijuana's administration, we can be assured that little progress will be made on this issue.

At this point, it should become clear to the reader that simply being a patient at an MMT clinic can be quite a tightrope-walk as the patient is forced to navigate the sometimes onerous and seemingly capricious clinic rules and regulations that must be adhered to, as well as the extreme deference they must pay to clinic directors and counselors, just in order to remain in good standing at their clinics.

As MMT patients, they can do nothing that might jeopardize their good standing, and this is subtly reinforced by reminders in the form of notices posted in various open areas of the clinic, usually reminding the patient that certain behaviors can be grounds for immediate termination, etc.

If much of this seems like unnecessary "hoop jumping," it's because it is. The vast majority of what is required by an MMT clinic of its patients is simply required because of federal regulations. The net result of many of these requirements is the effective infantilization of the MMT patient, a hand-coddling experience from door-to-door that can be deeply unsettling to an otherwise reasonable adult simply seeking medical care for a disease they cannot cure themselves.

There are an assortment of other *potential* difficulties with any given MMT provider that would fall under the miscellaneous category; whether clinic hours is one of them depends on one's individual time constraints as a patient. For some people, any clinic will invariably have convenient hours, but for many, some clinics with restricted hours can become problematic, particularly for those with steady employment. This appears to be one of the most difficult issues for the aforementioned patient group to deal with as most employers in the U.S. are quite limited in their ability to be "flexible."

The only permanent solution to this would be something known as Office Based Opioid Treatment (OBOT), an idea that will most likely never be implemented on any wide-scale basis. As it now stands, OBOT is implemented in the rarest of cases, at least partially because so many regulatory exceptions must be made just for one patient. The idea is simple enough; once a patient is stabilized on their methadone dose and all else is going well, their care would be taken over by a specially trained primary care physician who would see the MMT patient perhaps once a month and dispense the methadone via a standard monthly prescription which could be filled at any pharmacy, just as methadone is prescribed and dispensed for the treatment of pain. [60]

Though such physician-based advocacy groups such as ASAM (American Society for Addiction Medicine) have long advocated for a wide roll-out of such programs, there is still far too much stigma and re-sistance in the medical profession for OBOT to be widely implemented. In addition, the federal regulations as they now stand simply make it too prohibitive for easy implementation of OBOT, as they were designed en-tirely around the very concept of "separate but equal" medical care to be administered at MMT clinics.

Some patients can become so frustrated with a clinic's "tentacles" that they somewhat understandably act-out at any available clinic staff. It should come as little surprise that some patients are at their worst when they are infantilized in such a manner. Many otherwise normal people, when faced with punitive or infantalizing micromanagement will simply rise (or sink) to the level of behavior which is expected of them.

Saving the most controversial requirement of patients for last, the fol-lowing stipulation in the federal regulations can make for some serious headaches depending, once again, upon the clinic one attends;

"5.i. OTPs must provide adequate substance abuse counseling to each patient as clinically necessary. This counseling shall be provided by a program counselor, qualified by education, training, or experience to assess the psychological and sociological background of patients, to contribute to the appropriate treatment plan for the patient and to monitor patient prog-ress." (Appendix I)

This potential requirement for individualized counseling can serve as a tremendous source of headaches for the individual MMT patient, as every-thing from group attendance to one-on-one sessions with a counselor may be required, and these activities all take-up precious time that most recov-ering people would prefer to spend on more pedestrian activities, such as employment and caring for their families.

Again, this requirement can mean different things at different clin-ics, so if one has a problem with an excessive amount of counseling required of them by clinic protocols, it is incumbent upon them to talk with their counselor first and ask what their particular options are, since it is not unheard of for clinics to modify this requirement accordingly *depending upon* how well one is doing in their methadone maintenance treatment.

If after speaking to ones counselor nothing has changed, it is suggested that one go to the program's medical director and make their case personally to them, always bearing in mind that *they* have to bring something positive with respect to their treatment progress to the negotiation table. If nothing gives after having followed all the protocols of ones clinic, then the only other suggestion is to seek out another, more reasonable clinic. They are out there, though they can be hard to find.

Yes, there can be much excess baggage associated with methadone maintenance treatment depending on where one is geographically located. A closing word of advice to all *potential* MMT patients is that a "bad" MMT program is still better than none when one considers the potentially lethal alternatives.

9

THE FAILED WAR ON DRUGS (1909 TO PRESENT DAY)

The Failed War on Drugs has failed so miserably because of the Federal Government's insistence on primarily employing three failed methods to prosecute this "War." These, in turn, are based on false presumptions about the actual consequences of drug use. The three methods are interdiction, which is preventing drugs from entering the United States from other countries, secondly through a systematic campaign of directed misinformation, or what can more accurately be called propaganda, and thirdly through draconian prosecution.

For those who would take umbrage at the use of the word propaganda in describing the federal government's disinformation campaign, let us not forget that propaganda is simply the selective use of disinformation to attempt to influence a mass audience in a predetermined manner. Repeated often enough and for long enough, it becomes part of conventional wisdom. This happens to most accurately describe the public service announcements about drugs to a tee. [23]

Arguably the first shot fired across the bow in the WOD was the Federal Smoking Opium Exclusion Act of 1909, which outlawed the importation and use of opium. Close on its heels was the 1914 Harrison Narcotics Act which made both opioids and cocaine prescription-only medicines. The creation of the archetype/stereotype that we know today as a "junkie" had its roots in these legislative acts. [20,23]

After enactment of the Harrison Narcotics Act (1914) we began to see the cyclical and continuous repetition of overreaction and hysteria in response to a problem that, when viewed from an absolutely objective standpoint, did not merit the degree of alarm with which the press presented it, that being as a *calamitous crisis*.

The press addressed the issue in the manner that was customary of the day and age by seizing upon the most salacious aspects of the story, and in order to increase sales, they created for their readers the concept of the uncontrollable "junkie." Their portrayal of opioid addicted individuals was that of incorrigible individuals who could not be rehabilitated. They made a less than generous distinction as to kind and type. The first type was considered a "normal addict" who, in other words, received opioids iatrogenically and thereafter incidentally developed a habit. This "type" of individual was in the minority. [20]

The second type of individual, which made for far greater copy and sales, was presented to the public as the psychopathic "junkie" who was openly portrayed as fundamentally a deviant individual given to uncontrollable hedonistic impulses to such an extent that they were willing to commit heinous crimes and forsake both family bonds and social ties in order to get what they wanted. [20,23]

They defined the perceived deviant "junkie" as acting utterly without any kind of moral fiber. It is this latter "addict" that sold the most papers by appealing to readers prurient interests in the perceived and alien "other." As the decades progressed with no counterpoint to this disturbing stereotype, Hollywood took up the mantle of the deviant individual and made him a fixture of many Hollywood films such as The Man with the Golden Arm, Toxic Love, Candy, and Trainspotting, among many others.

De facto marijuana Prohibition began in earnest in 1939, when the then-mayor of New York City, Fiorello LaGuardia assembled a commission to investigate all aspects of marijuana consumption by city residents. Published in 1944, the report produced remarkably objective and frank investigative findings about the relative *harmlessness* of Cannabis smoking, and as such it inflamed the racist passions of the (now) infamous Harry Anslinger, who was the first commissioner of the Treasury Department's Bureau of Narcotics.

67

Anslinger, who can best be described as a man who possessed such animosity for all drugs that he would do anything in order to further his agenda of total prohibition, was infuriated by the release of the LaGuardia Commission report. It is no exaggeration to say that the prohibition of Cannabis in the U.S. was due almost single-handedly to Harry Anslinger. That he was a powerful man who knew how to bend federal legislators to do his bidding would be an understatement.

A poignant example of Anslinger's astonishing power over Washington, D.C. is best illustrated by the following excerpt.

"(Senator Joseph) McCarthy had also become addicted to morphine. Harry J. Anslinger, head of the Federal Bureau of Narcotics, became aware of McCarthy's addiction in the 1950s, and demanded he stop using the drug. McCarthy refused. In Anslinger's memoir, *The Murderers*, McCarthy is anonymously quoted as saying:

> I wouldn't try to do anything about it, Commissioner ... It will be
> the worse for you ... and if it winds up in a public scandal and that
> should hurt this country, I wouldn't care [...] The choice is yours.

Anslinger decided to give McCarthy access to morphine in secret from a pharmacy in Washington, DC. The morphine was paid for by the Federal Bureau of Narcotics, right up to McCarthy's death. Anslinger never publicly named McCarthy, and he threatened, with prison, a journalist who uncovered the story. However, McCarthy's identity was known to Anslinger's agents, and journalist Maxine Cheshire confirmed his identity with Will Oursler, co-author of *The Murderers*, in 1978." [23]

Having been active in the federal enforcement of alcohol prohibition before moving on to the Bureau of Narcotics, he not only had an incredible amount of animus towards all drugs, but to marijuana in particular, which he insisted was due to his (erroneous) belief that marijuana was, "the gateway to all other drugs." This has been widely and repeatedly disproven, both anecdotally and by controlled clinical studies. [48]

The propaganda employed at the time by the Bureau of Narcotics was very effective because to this very day, a substantial minority of the American population continues to believe that marijuana is an *intrinsically dangerous* and "immoral" drug that plants users feet on the pathway to all other manner of addictions, even when confronted with *all objective evidence to the contrary.* [48]

That Harry Anslinger ensured the prohibition of psychoactive drugs in the U.S. is a rather well known fact. What is less well know is that he also single-handedly *dictated drug policy to the rest of the world*, via his appointment to the U.N. after retiring from the bureau.

Though many countries in 1960 objected to the strong-arm tactics Anslinger used to achieve absolute prohibition, few at the time had any real power to resist, as there were many inter-dependent financial relationships between U.N. member countries and the U.S. which Anslinger leveraged to the fullest extent in order to achieve his ends. [23,61]

At first, many countries such as Bolivia and India, resisted, stating that certain substance use was particular to the practice of their culture. Anslinger would, however, have none of it. The more they objected to falling in line with the U.S.'s drug policy goals, the more Anslinger reminded them that the U.S. *could* withdraw its subsidies, should they persist in their resistance. Pretty soon, all countries fell into line. [23]

As a result, the Single Convention on Narcotic Drugs of 1961 was passed, a document to which all relevant nations were signatories. In this Convention, Cannabis, coca, and opioids were the drugs being controlled, but the agreement laid the further groundwork for The Convention on Psychotropic Substances of 1971 which further broadened the legal reach of the treaty to include *all* psychoactive substances such as amphetamines, barbiturates, hallucinogens, etc.

Put simply, the world-wide prohibitionary stance on psychoactive substances had its genesis and continued staying power as the *singular result* of U.S. foreign policy against the member nations of the U.N. [23] To say that many countries were and continue to be strong-armed into punitive, prohibitionist policies is not an exaggeration, and this is best attested to by the fact that U.N. member nations have now formed their own think-tanks that regard the WOD as a failure, the best representative of those agencies being the Global Commission on Drug Policy (www.globalcommissionon-drugs.org). Their approach, embodied in their numerous position papers, is a total rejection of the WOD and of the disaster that it has wrought.

The fact that the entire world's drug control policy has its origins with one man, Harry Anslinger, might go a good way towards explaining *why* the WOD has been *such* a disastrous failure. Unbeknownst to many, Anslinger's hatred of drugs paralleled his hatred of all non-Caucasians, and his early scare campaigns, consisting of well-placed "news" stories in the papers of the day, were blatantly racist in their themes and undertones. The fact that he was a racist had a tremendous bearing on how everything con-current to the WOD unfolded, since Anslinger was well aware of the racial animus and fears held by the general Caucasian population of the time. As can be seen from the headlines and stories of that time, he shrewdly inter-twined the two topics in a shamelessly inflammatory manner that today would be known as "race baiting." [61]

To this day, a disproportionate percentage of dark-skinned minorities receive the brunt of criminal prosecution for drug offenses, and this is in light of the fact that more white people consume psychoactive drugs than do minorities. To say that current drug policies may be somewhat of a proxy for "racial" policy is probably not popular, but it is most reflective of the current realities of race-relations in America. [20,23,65]

Another factor at play that must be addressed as being equally important in establishing the creation of the "junkie" archetype in the United states is intimately tied to the evolution of the medical industry, specifically, the role that was played by the then-young American Medical Association (AMA) as they initially attempted to address and treat drug addiction in response to mounting public, and subsequently political, pressures.

Here we see history repeating itself in both the extent to which the repetition is occurring, and the reasons for its recurrence. At the turn of the last century, physicians were still in their proverbial infancy (particularly within the newborn field of psychiatry) with respect to the levels of power, privilege and control over their profession that they enjoy today, and the physician's concern at that time was first and foremost with achieving a legitimate professional status as a rigid scientific discipline. [20]

Wherever humans are, there will always be those individuals who behave as though they possess little conscience, and members of the medical profession have proved to be no exception to this axiom. There will always be medical doctors who may not possess the most integrated personalities or practice with professional objectivity.

The experts of the early 20th century were no exception, and many had barely more of a clue as to what they were doing than the people whom they were attempting to treat. [20] At the time, one data point that most physicians of all disciplines agreed upon was that the vast majority of addicted individuals that they treated were morally degenerate people who were not worthy of much effort on the part of the medical profession. Of the rest that perhaps came from a similar socioeconomic background as the physician himself or who had perhaps acquired their addiction iatrogenically, the treatment protocol and judicial repercussions would often be mitigated. [20] This is another example of how the more things change, the more they stay the same.

The main reason that such a heavy emphasis was placed on the addicted individuals morality and character was because at that point in time, psychiatry was at the peak of its' obsession with Freudian-based psychoanalytic concepts like oral fixation, anal fixation, the Oedipus complex, penis envy, etc. That the psychiatric profession would continue to lose another fifty years on what we now know to be totally *ineffective psychoanalysis* was something that simply had to occur historically in order for the profession to develop more legitimate, evidence-based treatments.

The Harrison Narcotics Act of 1914 did contain a loophole that allowed physicians to prescribe morphine to already addicted/dependent patients. That grace period lasted for approximately five years at which point physicians began to be portrayed by the media as dope pushers and enablers, not only serving as a part of the problem but as the *root cause* of the problem, for as conventional wisdom went, without a prescription for pain medication an addicted individual would not be created.

Around 1930, Anslinger, in complete disregard of the fact that they were operating legally, had thousands of morphine "maintenance" clinics shut down and had physicians across the U.S. arrested, with many being sentenced to periods of incarceration for having done nothing more than *legally* help addicted individuals. [23] This is a large part of the reason why, to this day, physicians may not legally prescribe an opioid to a *known* addicted individual unless it is for the control of severe pain, and it is also why methadone may not be prescribed by ordinary physicians through a pharmacy for the treatment of addicted individuals, but instead may only be dispensed by a federally licensed Opioid Treatment Program (OTP.)

After the shuttering of the last morphine clinic, the black-market for narcotics in general *exploded*, with opioids being the most consistently desired product. From the 1930's until roughly 1970, American opioid addicts were left to fend entirely for themselves. As mentioned before, there were the federal Narcotic Farms in Kentucky and Texas after circa 1935, but these were little more than federally-run withdrawal hospitals with some patients being remanded there by the courts, and others being there voluntarily. Because of their abysmal "success" rates, the last farm was converted into a prison in 1974.

Fast forward to June 18, 1971. It is not a coincidence that the The Convention on Psychotropic Substances of 1971 was ratified by the U.N. in this seminal year. After having released a special report to Congress the previous day in which Richard Nixon asserted that drug use was "public enemy number one," Nixon went before the press and publicly declared that he was declaring a "War on Drugs." He began to prosecute this war by, not surprisingly, going after interdiction, unleashing an aggressive pro-paganda campaign and, of course, constantly referencing the "get tough" on users/dealers rhetoric.

If this reads like history repeating itself, it absolutely is. The War on Drugs of the 21st Century is, in its methods and techniques, no different than the War on Drugs of 1971. Parenthetically speaking, Nixon himself was a notorious bigot, at best, who also ruthlessly exploited white fear of minorities by utilizing Patrick Buchanan's infamous "Southern Strategy." Race has never left the WOD equation.

Nixon began marshaling his troops by enlisting the help of celebri-ties, the most notable being "the King" himself, Elvis Presley, whom he deputized as an honorary DEA Agent. Of course, Elvis Presley's image had tremendous advertising potential, and this was not lost on Nixon. As Nixon's message of, "all drugs = bad drugs" worked its way into the popular culture, America began to see the aggressive prosecution of primarily dark skinned Americans whose only crime was to have an opioid habit or to simply have been a consumer of marijuana or some other drug while having been unlucky enough to get caught holding.

The "mash-up" of all drugs into one amorphous jumble only served, in reality, to *conflate all drugs with one another*. Since, according to the DEA, marijuana fell under the same schedule as did heroin, there was an *implied equivalency*, and thus the prohibitionists were very well served by this obfuscation as they began to point out that since marijuana was on the same schedule as heroin, it must be equally "bad," toxic, and addictive as the much harder drugs on that schedule. That these tactics were not only unhelpful but actually *counterproductive* is something that the DEA has, according to its scheduling, never acknowledged nor changed since 1970. Importantly, it must be noted here that all of the classic *psychedelics* such as LSD, psilocybin and mescaline were also included in Schedule I of the Controlled Substances Act (or CSA) of 1970.

Most Americans of a particular age can remember the absurd Public Service Announcements (or PSAs) from the 1980's which advised children that smoking a joint was equivalent to frying ones brain in a frying pan. It was exactly these kinds of dramatic equivocations that, more than anything else, turned off an entire generation to the Just Say No message, for, "if the government was lying about marijuana, so too was it lying about other drugs, cocaine in particular."

Arguably the tactics that first began with Anslinger, continued under Nixon and Reagan, and persist to this day serve to only *worsen* the drug problem, as any astute observer can attest to. This is because when people started out casually using marijuana after their foray into the world of cigarette smoking (which is the actual, proven gateway drug), and realized that all of the egregious harms that they were warned about did not come to pass, they falsely *presumed* that since the warnings about marijuana were a lie, then the warnings about other drugs must at a minimum be overstated or at worst also be lies. [48]

And so it came to pass that of the pot smokers who would never have tried cocaine when it became popular starting in the mid 1970s, a sizable number decided to try their hand at this "new" drug called cocaine, to sometimes disastrous effect.

A point very worth mentioning here is that had marijuana been legalized or at least not criminalized, people's contact with the criminal underworld would have been greatly reduced, which in turn would have meant that the average citizen would have had far less environmental exposure to these potentially more dangerous hard drugs. As we recall from earlier in this text, ones environment is at least half of the necessary equation for opioid addiction to take root.

Stigmatization about drug use is a natural, if malignant, outgrowth of the contempt with which the federal government has treated the truth about drugs. And what is further clear is that whole generations were sold a fake bill of goods with respect to information about psychoactive drugs, so it should come as little surprise now that the stigma attached to addiction is so brutal and complete, because it has been based largely on a disinformation campaign that has been conducted over multiple decades.

If a 25 year old neurotypical person bears a strong stigma against opioid addicted individuals, it is most likely because from their perspective, that is how it's always been: their grandparents railed against drugs (thanks to Anslinger and his generation), their parents railed against drugs (thanks to Nixon, and then Reagan), so why would they have any other attitude towards the afflicted except hostility and fear based on stigma, without the modulating impact of factual information and empathy?

The leviathan that is now the American pharmaceutical industry was born at the turn of the last century and has in the last two decades of the 21st century taken on a life of its own. Though it should have no business in the development of care plans for recovery and healing, it instead has taken a foremost role in the decision making guidelines, displacing the patient as an incidental object, relegating him into the role of a minor actor as to whether or not said patient will be properly treated. Because of the for-profit model which is unique to American medicine, whether or not someone gets a life-saving drug or not can be entirely determined by their ability to pay the exorbitant prices for it that have been predetermined by the drug's manufacturer. Even generic drugs are becoming prohibitively expensive. Why is the federal government not declaring "war" on the pharmaceutical industry who are responsible for the extortionary drug pricing that is being exacted against Americans?

Just before the turn of this century, Purdue Pharma came up with a scheme whereby they took a 100-year old opiate (oxycodone) and by simply changing it into a unique, time-release formulation (OxyContin) that avoided the problems encountered with serum peaks and troughs, they then cleverly marketed this massively powerful opioid through a public relations campaign unlike anything before it to individual hospitals, physicians and researchers. They sponsored researchers that "confirmed" Purdue's exuberant and unfounded claims that this form of oxycodone was far less addictive than other forms of the medication. Of course, they priced it far above its actual added value, with each dosage unit being made for under one dollar, yet being priced to earn them *thousands of percent* in profit.

Before, physicians had been operating under the model of extreme reticence in prescribing these medications. For reasons that will forever remain relatively opaque, physicians who *should* have known better were fooled into thinking that OxyContin was no more addictive than Darvon, with sometimes disastrous results. One crucial point to remember here is that while physicians and Purdue pharma didn't create the opioid epidemic, they certainly did their part by making these Schedule II opioid medications much more widely available for even the smallest aches and pains. Like the federal governments' response to the medical community in the years that followed passage of the Harrison Narcotics Act in the second decade of the 20th Century, the DEA is once again barking up the wrong tree in prosecuting physicians who continue to prescribe pain medication for legacy chronic pain patients. (see Chapter 10)

Important to remember at this point is how often grandstanding politicians will utilize the "opioid crisis" to manipulate their constituents, except when their constituent's children are themselves afflicted. For example, only recently have we seen the expansion of the opioid treatment discussion branch out to Medication Assisted Treatment or MAT, something that would have been unheard of twenty years ago when all that was sincerely offered was abstinence based treatment. And yet, as long as the people dying were mostly poor and dark-skinned, these disastrous results were considered acceptable. Only when white, suburban youth and their white family, friends and neighbors began to develop addictions and die from overdosing was there a resumption of serious discussion about MAT, since abstinence-based treatment providers have been unsuccessful at keeping opioid addicted individuals sober, let alone alive. [8,42]

Again, it bears reemphasizing here that MAT, particularly in the form of Methadone Maintenance Treatment or MMT, has been the most studied and proven effective treatment modality for the last 50 years, so the information itself is far from new. [8,29,42] What is new is the political and civic will, born of desperation, to see it through and help it vastly expand its current treatment population.

As concerns interdiction, the War on Drugs has been an abject and predictable failure. One need only look at the nearly 4000 miles of our contiguous borders with Canada and Mexico as well as our vast expanses of ocean front borders to draw the same conclusion. If interdiction has been an utter failure in countries as small and easily controllable as the Netherlands, which possesses only 919 miles of border, how could it possibly work in a nation like America, which is the size of a continent and which possess a population that is unmatched in both its desire for and consumption of all manner of drugs?

That the limits of interdiction have long ago been reached is evidenced by the increasing presence of drugs for sale on U.S. streets, plummeting prices, and an increasing assortment of drugs for sale. New players have entered the marketplace, one of the best examples being China. While China does not have any official policy of exporting addictive drugs to the United States, it nonetheless has a bustling organic chemical industry which has been commissioned by Westerners to produce all manner of illicit substances, arguably the most notorious being the fentanyls, for example carfentanil, 3-methyl-fentanyl, remifentanil, and lofentanil. This is by no means an exhaustive list of all the fentanyl analogs, of which there are potentially hundreds.

The fentanyls themselves pose a particular problem for interdiction for two main reasons. First, they are fully synthetic and thus do not require opioid precursors, but most importantly pertinent to this discussion is the fact that they are *astonishing* in their potency, so much so that for some versions of fentanyl analogs, one ounce of the fentanyl would be equivalent to several thousand pounds of heroin. A simple illustration is the fentanyl analog Carfentanil. *On a weight for weight basis*, one would need 10,000 times less Carfentanil than one would need morphine *to produce an equivalent effect.* The practical implications of this are stunning in that what used to require a truck load to conceal its contents now can be easily hidden inside a soda pop can.

As could be expected, the interdiction failures with respect to fentanyl analogs have been directly responsible for the soaring overdose rate in the U.S. This is the case precisely because the fentanyls are *so potent* that traditional drug dealers do not understand how to properly "cut/stomp" this deadly product in order to make it safe for consumption.

Interdiction itself appears to have two ineffective prongs. The first prong is our country's predilection for going to drug producing nations and telling them to stop manufacturing drugs, "or else," (usually, with the threatened cut-off of U.S. aid and/or trade,) and the second prong is to arrest individual users and small time dealers, people who are most often selling small quantities to support their own habits. This does *nothing* to interrupt the actual flow of, or demand for, these drugs. It only diverts valuable limited resources away from the actual effective work of discouraging the consumption of these drugs (that is provided by an honest education on the likely dangers), and properly treating citizens who have become addicted.

The third tine of the failed war on drugs (WOD) is the *criminalization of a disease*, since addicted individuals would not be prosecuted if they were viewed, first and foremost, as the medically ill individuals which they are. The "lawbreaking" aspect of this disease is utterly secondary and tangential to the disease itself, a direct by-product of the draconian laws surrounding opioid possession.

Alcohol maintains a special place in the pantheon of addictive substances in that in addition to destroying families and the communities in which they reside, it is also responsible on average for more than 88,000 fatalities, and *2.5 million years of potential life lost, every year.* Deaths which are, *de facto*, accepted without question, with society-at-large bearing the brunt of the staggering costs. About $2 of every $5 of the economic costs of excessive alcohol use are paid by federal, state, and local governments, and excessive alcohol consumption cost the United States $249 billion in 2010. [66]

The irony continues when we consider that *were* alcohol to be scheduled as a controlled substance by the DEA, it would *have to be* placed in Schedule II of the Controlled Substances Act. Schedule II is the most restrictive schedule and is reserved for drugs which, though they have a medical purpose, are considered to be so highly addictive that they must be more restricted than almost all other controlled substances. Some representative examples of medications in this schedule are amphetamines, cocaine, morphine, pentobarbital, secobarbital and amobarbital. It is not a coincidence that the last three drugs noted are all short-acting barbiturates, since the pharmacological action of this class of drugs is indistinguishable from the action of alcohol in the human brain.

Some readers might raise an objection regarding the negative effects of the prosecutorial aspect of the War on Drugs, claiming that courts are now increasingly steering drug offenders into "diversion" programs and treatment facilities and that, in fact, there are even specialized drug courts precisely for this purpose. To this it must be said that this jurisprudential approach is applied very arbitrarily and when it is applied, the final decisions rest only with the judge, not with the medical advice that that judge may very well hear. Said another way, a drug court judge can subjectively choose to ignore medical opinions and render at worst a punitive judgment, or at best a judgment which, though it is treatment based, and thus fundamentally well-meant, is nonetheless counterproductive because drug courts by a wide majority still prefer ineffectual abstinence-based programs, which for the vast majority of opioid addicted individuals act as nothing more than revolving doors into further morbidity and mortality.

It cannot go without saying that the current WOD claims hundreds of thousands of innocent lives every year. When we look just south of our border to Mexico, there is a body count of circa 70,000 innocent civilians, as of the latest count, who just happened to be in the wrong place at the wrong time. As a first-world nation that supposedly respects human rights, where does that leave us in terms of our collective humanity, or lack thereof? Lest we forget, the United States was one of the first signatories of the Geneva Convention on Basic Human Rights, and so it *appears* like the U.S. government is entirely accepting of all the *foreign* civilian carnage *in the name of saving lives here at home.* Yet, any thoughtful person can see that the aforementioned "equation" is hopelessly distorted towards a "shoot first, ask questions later" mind-set.

That the WOD has always had, and continues to have, an element of sadism to it might sound unreasonable, but this reality appears to exist everywhere one looks, from mass incarceration of opioid addicts to "boot camp" style therapeutic communities, there is much to be said about how poorly opioid addicted individuals are treated, not to mention the innocent civilians caught in the proverbial cross-fire.

Not forgetting that addicts (so far) cannot receive MAT in U.S. jails and prisons, cold turkey withdrawal is a form of cruel and unusual punishment that is exacted upon physically addicted individuals every day across the nation. There are a handful of cases going through the courts now that are trying desperately to change this but, as the saying goes, the wheels of justice turn slowly. It will probably be a good number of years until this systemic sadism is removed from our jurisprudential treatment of opioid addicts.

One of the perverse consequences of crude jail-house withdrawal is that, of those that survive it, they become many times as likely to overdose on discharge when compared to non-addicted inmates, and one of the stark realities of overdose is that not everyone survives. Said another way, forced withdrawal during incarceration results in *vastly* increased morbidity and mortality for those same inmates after release. [67,72]

A large part of the war on the WOD consists of removing these cruel punishments, encoded by the criminalization of opioid addiction, from our law books. That will be the easy part. The more difficult part will be removing the dreadful stigma from this severe addiction, as it has been 100 years in the making. Every day brings with it the chance to see things from a different perspective, so let's try and ensure that that chance begins today.

10

New CDC Guidelines
and The pain crisis

A brief reminder is in order here;

"The pain patient, whose remission of pain allows discontinuance of opiates, often requires treatment for opiate withdrawal symptoms. <u>*However, these patients usually manifest no compulsion or drug-seeking behavior.*</u> The treatment of pain patients who do not have a diagnosis or history of opiate addiction in the setting of a program designed for the treatment of opiate addiction is rarely appropriate. Such pain patients are more appropriately managed in the pain clinic or in a physician's office." [120] [ed. note: *emphasis added*)

In response to the opioid crisis in the U.S., the CDC has adopted non-binding guidelines for long-term (chronic) opioid treatment for medical professionals, but these "suggested" guidelines have turned out to be a *nightmare* for chronic pain patients, even those with cancer, since they have had a chilling-effect on physician prescribing of opioids to these patients (even long-term patients.) Particularly in light of the long-known fact that patients treated with opioids for severe pain rarely become addicted to them, this focus on chronic pain patients is, at the very least, misguided. The effects of this new focus on chronic pain patients have been undeniably harsh, and this mistreatment is the main reason for the necessity of this chapter.

There will *always* be a small number of people who are routinely prescribed and must indefinitely take opioids for chronic pain, and an even smaller number who are given opioids because they have a terminal illness that produces severe pain, for example, in a cancer patient whose tumor has metastasized to multiple organs.

It is unfortunate that the CDC is now *insisting* that there is *no evidence* for long-term effectiveness of opioids in chronic pain, when, in fact, there is a *universe* of anecdotal and empirical evidence (supplied by millions of chronic pain patients and their doctors) that they *do* work in the long-term for moderate-to-severe chronic pain. These poor souls have done nothing wrong, and yet *they* are now being punished for an epidemic of opioid overdose deaths which are now due, by a wide margin, to illicit opioids like heroin. Chronic pain patients with legitimate pain issues are not, for the most part, part of the problem, and they need to be left alone and given back their quality-of-life-saving medications.

In the interim, these guidelines have done *remarkably little* to reduce opioid abuse or deaths, which for years now have been due, by far, much more to heroin and illicit fentanyl than to prescription opioids. The media itself has done nothing to help this situation and has gone a long way towards making it worse, since they are perpetuating the CDC's misleading statistics. [121]

What they *have* done is caused suicides among legitimate chronic pain patients (even veterans) *forcibly weaned* off of their legal opioids, or caused equally desperate pain patients to seek-out illegal opioids; in either case, the result is equally tragic, since the CDC guidelines actually *directly contribute* to the rapid increase in deaths from illicit opioids, and do nothing (literally nothing) to save patient's lives. [118,124,125]

In point of fact, the guidelines are nothing less than cruelly arbitrary and wholly ineffective for chronic pain patients, and even hospitalized patients in acute, e.g. post-surgical pain. If the pendulum swung too far from the late 90's until circa 2012, it has now *barbarically* swung in the opposite direction, *to no ones benefit*. Under-treatment of the most severe pain is now rampant in the U.S.. [26,114,115,146]

A lesser known fact about the guidelines is that they were suggested by a group calling themselves, "Physicians for Responsible Opioid

Prescribing," a group consisting neither entirely of pain specialists or even regular physicians: Instead, professionals with *obvious conflicts of interest* also participated in the design of the guidelines, particularly acupuncturists, naturopaths, and chiropractors. [122] Too convoluted to elaborate upon here, I left the guidelines themselves for Appendix IV.

As it turned out, 2010 was a watershed year not only in terms of opioid overdoses, but especially with respect to overdoses caused by heroin. It is not a coincidence that 2010 was the year that Purdue Pharma (the manufacturers of OxyContin,) introduced a reformulated, tamper-proof version of the drug. This formulation effectively prevented a person from crushing the tablet in order to snort it or inject it, rendering it usable only orally. We see that from 2010 onwards, deaths by heroin increased by 500%. At the same time, we also observed a rising *"consumption pattern"* (as opposed to overdoses) for all other opioids *except* methadone (more solid evidence that methadone itself has little to no "street value.")

Once OxyContin was no longer abusable, consumption of all other opioids increased because the addicted people were simply moving on to the *next available opioid*. The connection between the reformulation of OxyContin and the increased use of and death by heroin is one that is not simple conjecture, but has actually been posited by respected medical journals, and it goes as follows: with the reformulation of OxyContin, those users who had been abusing OxyContin intravenously or intranasally, being no longer able to get their drug of choice, resorted to purchasing heroin to replace that drug. [123]

Unfortunately, with heroin come all of the problems associated with its illegality: impurities, unknown amendments, imprecise dosage, etc. Individuals now at the mercy of what little information drug dealers could provide them with ended up dead on bathroom stall floors, most likely because they had been used to a standardized and precise dosage with pre-reformulation OxyContin, and carried that assumption over to their use of heroin. [67,72]

What has also been pointed out in the medical journals is that since 2010, the rates of Hepatitis C infection have begun to climb again after a period of stabilization, and it is surmised that this is due to needle sharing which is common for heroin users to resort to for lack of easily available *sterile* injection paraphernalia. Across America, a total lack of monitored injection facilities and a dearth of needle exchange programs has only added fuel to the Hepatitis C (and HIV) fire. [63]

This is how we have lost a generation of sons and daughters. To further complicate matters, the heroin overdoses are increasingly often turning out to be, upon closer inspection, fentanyl overdoses. What is crucial to remember at this juncture is that we are not speaking of pharmaceutical, prescribed fentanyl, but rather synthetic analogs that have been manufactured illicitly, most of which is accomplished in China.

In 2016 after a steady and steep uptick in opioid deaths beginning in the year 2010, the Centers for Disease Control (CDC) issued guidelines for prescribing opioids for both acute and chronic pain. The guidelines are relatively self explanatory to anyone who has had proper pharmacological training, and *most* of the recommendations do not pose any adverse consequence to chronic pain patients.

This being said, there are some serious sticking points in the recommendations that have caused a literal outcry amongst chronic pain patients and their physicians across the nation. These sticking points have to do with what the guidelines state should be both the maximal daily dosage of opioids, as well as stating what the length of time of opioid administration should be. [115]

Even though the CDC guidelines are non-binding and are only "suggestions" made to clinicians, in reality, they have had a deeply chilling effect across the country among medical practitioners of every stripe with respect to their treatment of both acute and chronic pain. The reason for this chilling effect is because the Drug Enforcement Administration (DEA) is concurrently and aggressively pursuing physicians in an arbitrary manner for over-prescription of opioids, the problem arising mainly from the arbitrary character of their selection criteria. Said another way, no physician has any clue as to what would cause the DEA to visit *their* practice for a spontaneous audit that could lead to anything from loss of prescribing privileges to loss of licensure, up to and including criminal prosecution. [146]

As if this were not problematic enough, even though the guidelines wisely suggest that in certain situations clinicians should consider offering naloxone along with the opioid prescription (naloxone is an opioid antagonist administered to patients in case of overdose), in reality, a very high percentage of clinicians are *absolutely* against providing a prescription for naloxone with an opioid prescription. This is because some physicians feel that it is a "get out of jail free card" for the patient, essentially sending the message that with naloxone in hand, the patient would throw caution to the wind and not exactly follow the directions provided with the opioid prescription. Other physicians may proffer slightly different reasons for not providing naloxone co-prescriptions, but they all share in common a concern about what kind of "message this would send" to the patient. As is demonstrated in chapter 19, most physicians are very biased against opioid addicted individuals.

It is important to remember that in the discussion revolving around opioids, we must address *all* aspects of opioid use and administration, and no where is this more acutely felt than with chronic pain patients right now. A simple Google search will reveal endless horror stories of pain patients who have been unceremoniously "tossed to the wolves" as their physicians have either drastically reduced their pain medication or discontinued it altogether. [18,113-115,146]

The real world effects of these guidelines have been *devastating* to chronic pain patients to a degree which *cannot be overstated.* Since the release of the guidelines, a majority of chronic pain patients have found themselves at the losing end of a battle between their physicians, their pharmacists and the their insurance providers. [146]

Minor inconveniences are not what are being referenced here, what we are addressing is the reality that an unknown number of chronic pain patients have resorted to everything from going to the streets to procure illicit opioids up to taking their lives to escape the unrelenting pain their conditions condemn them to. [124,125]

What has brought them to this point is that *even pain specialists* are now increasingly seeking to reduce the daily dosage that chronic pain patients have been on for years, if not to out and out discontinue the medication entirely. No chronic pain patient is unaffected, that includes patients with cancer pain. Oddly enough, pain patients are now being treated as "known" opioid addicts, a.k.a. being "presumed guilty until proven innocent," and this is irrespective of what their medical records (i.e. history) have objectively recorded over the years. The pendulum has swung so far that physicians have so acutely come to fear the loss of their livelihoods that they are now actively abandoning the Hippocratic Oath that guided their practice of medicine for years. Close on the heels of abandoning their oath, they are abandoning their patients. [18,124] This is an unacceptable state of affairs.

Slowly and cautiously, physicians are beginning to speak out against the ridiculously restrictive CDC guidelines. That they are doing so very carefully is understandable (to a degree) in light of the para-militarization of the DEA. The DEA is taking actions that should not be their purview, in particular, threatening physicians with revocation of their DEA licenses to prescribe controlled substances. Even though controlled substances make up only a small portion of all prescriptions, a physician is essentially without prescribing ability without their DEA license, since controlled substances ultimately make-up an important part of a physicians pharmacopoeia. Perhaps stated dramatically, the DEA currently has the power of life-and-death over a physicians career (and a civilian's freedom,) and this is too much power, concentrated in too few hands. [26, 113,115,119,146]

The fear of the DEA is so great that it is destroying many doctor-patient relationships, not to mention patients' quality of life. We would be remiss not to mention that this overarching fear of the DEA is spreading into all aspects of prescribing *any* controlled medications. Even medications as innocuous as sleeping medications like Schedule IV Ambien (zolpidem tartrate) are now being treated like Schedule II medications, requiring some patients to have to visit their doctors offices to pick up a new prescription on a monthly basis, whereas before a simple call to the pharmacy by the doctor could procure them a prescription with up to 5 refills. It appears as if what was once an imperfect system has been rendered utterly broken. [146]

If some of this sounds familiar, it is for good reason. What we are seeing today is essentially a repetition of what happened in the late 1920s as the newly formed Bureau of Narcotics aggressively pursued and prosecuted thousands of doctors across the country for having committed the "crime" of prescribing opioids to addicted individuals. [121,124] That the physicians were doing so was based entirely upon the fact that the 1914 Harrison Narcotic Act contained a loophole which *allowed* physicians to legally continue prescribing opioids to known addicted individuals, said another way, this was the earliest form of maintenance treatment.

That this treatment modality did not last was due to the vast overreach of, once again, Harry Anslinger. It mattered little to him whether what the doctors were doing was legal or not: he was not having any of it on his watch. Under his direction, he sent narcotics agents to all corners of the country to dragnet these physicians who were *legally* prescribing opioids for addicted individuals. It would be fair to say that all of the physicians caught in this dragnet had their livelihoods destroyed. Not only with the loss of licensure, but often also with lengthy prison sentences. That the courts saw no contradiction in Anslinger's disregard for the law was a powerful indicator of how rapidly his anti-drug hysteria had metastasized to the general public, so that few people were willing to openly argue in defense of these physicians, and of those that did, they did so at their own peril. [23]

To prevent history from repeating itself, it is crucial that we now begin a *new discussion* that is based on clinical facts and established medical research as opposed to clinging to the same old tropes and memes which have been put forth by the media, our government, and religious institutions who, dominating public discourse, have created *manufactured consent*.

Manufactured consent, in this context, is the concept that large swaths of the public can be made to agree upon a given narrative, indeed almost any narrative, if that narrative is established by authoritative institutions and then *endlessly repeated*. Joseph Goebbels is a historical example of someone who understood this and, very cynically, utilized it to great effect to "move the masses". This says nothing about the veracity of the narrative, which is why it is referred to as *manufactured* consent.

The information that has come out in the last 20 years alone would easily suffice for a total revision of the dominant narrative which insists, among other things, that abstinence is the ***only*** answer to opioid addiction and that anything less than this benchmark is tantamount to "capitulation."

This theme of capitulation appears again and again when we see, for example, harm reduction activists attempting to start needle exchange programs in their communities in order to prevent loss of life through the spread of HIV and Hepatitis C, among other diseases, to members of the drug injecting community. That addiction has nothing to do with capitulation is only possible when it is viewed through objective, clinical eyes, and not through the distorted lens of moral judgment.

The solution to this problem is so simple that it strains credulity as to why it has not been implemented, and that would be for the CDC to update their guidelines and do so in a manner that is consistent with good patient care, which holds paramount the alleviation of suffering. This, coupled with the demilitarization of the DEA as it relates to doctor-patient relationships, would restore our nation to a position of strength and health which it currently does not have.

Additional necessary changes would involve creating systems of accountability among healthcare workers that would strongly disincentivize the use of any form of derogatory language when speaking of addicted patients or patients on MMT. [18] One of the best ways that this could occur would be if physicians would be personally introduced to stabilized long-term MMT patients, preferably in a lecture/question & answer format. This would do wonders towards wiping away the ugly stereotypes of anybody involved with opioids, as physicians might realize that they have much more in common with the hated 'other' than they do differences. [18]

Perhaps most controversially, it would involve the CDC doing a complete re-calculation and re-ordering of the causes of opioid overdose deaths in the U.S., and doing so would involve first admitting that the overdose crisis is *not* being fueled primarily by legitimately prescribed opioids, but rather by illicit black-market opioids. Starting in 2010, we saw a strong uptick in the number of opioid overdoses due to heroin, but at the same time, a decrease in overdoses due to legitimate pain medications. This trend has continued through to today.

Real, patient-centered reform would also involve the CDC clarifying that the sharp rise in heroin overdoses is in large part due to their contamination with ultra-powerful fentanyl analogs. Stated another way, the CDC would be most wise in altogether backing down from their 2016 guidelines, as these do nothing but hurt legitimate pain patients, and they *do nothing to stop the precipitous rise in overdoses.*

Most people are fortunate enough to never have to suffer from excruciating, unending, debilitating pain. One would hope that most people can discuss this issue with a calm demeanor and hard facts in hand, because as of right now, both of these are missing from the greater opioid debate. To attempt to empathize with someone who has such brutal pain issues that without opioid medications they would be very seriously suicidal takes a certain degree of willingness to imagine the unimaginable. It cannot be denied that now is a time when average, neurotypical people *need* to be able to discuss this very issue without resorting to demagoguery, and this is one issue that tends to lend itself easily to simplistic demagoguery.

Imagine, for a moment, that your loved one suffered from such severe, intractable pain that *nothing* besides opioids could make life livable again. Would you yourself personally deny them relief? The question, of course, is rhetorical, but it is designed to get people thinking about what they would do were *they* in a position of control over opioid dispensing, and whether it ultimately is good public-health policy to keep increasing the difficulty that patients experience should they require opioids. [146]

We would be remiss to not mention the crisis of pain that is affecting the vast majority of people on this globe, the most by far in Africa.

"In Senegal the average patient who needs it gets *13 mg of morphine a year*, compared with *55,704 mg in America*. *Across sub-Saharan Africa nine-tenths of cancer sufferers in moderate or severe pain die without the relief granted by opioids*...The morphine shortage stems from bad policies. In the 1980s and 1990s, as part of its "war on drugs", America cut aid and imposed sanctions on countries that were not tough enough on trafficking. It listed Nigeria as uncooperative from 1994 to 1998 (during a criminal dictatorship), suspended military aid and blocked loans....There is little threat of being penalized today. But taboos about opioid use, restrictions on prescriptions and import barriers are still in place across much of Africa, says Barbara Goedde at the Global Commission on Drug Policy. *In 2012, although some 200,000 Nigerians died of AIDS-related causes, often in severe pain,* the country imported no morphine and said there was no need for it." [119] [ed. note: *emphases added*]

At this point in the discussion we would do well to remember that Africa and the rest of the under-developed world's nations have the destructive drug policies that they do only because of Harry Anslinger, who single-handedly orchestrated American hegemony at the U.N. regarding world drug control. [23] For no other reason than continued intense financial (and military) pressure by the U.S.A. are these policies still being followed, and the suffering thereby created has been unimaginable. Most humans wouldn't treat animals so poorly, so why are we treating other humans so mercilessly?

In the midst of all the current hysteria over opioid addiction, we would also do well to remember that opium itself has been with us since the dawn of mankind. Most other civilizations found reasonable ways to deal with the "opium question" when confronted with it: It's is time we took some lessons from history, making it a point to ignore the disastrous lessons that have characterized the last hundred years regarding this issue. [20]

11

THE DIFFERENCE BETWEEN ADDICTION AND DEPENDENCE/ PSEUDO-ADDICTION

Understanding the differences between addiction, dependence and pseudo-addiction is critical if one is to be able to fully discuss this topic. It is critical that these distinctions are drawn in order to ensure that the differences are crystal clear, for without this clarity we can't even know what it is we are trying to treat. In the age of social media and the 24 hour news cycle, the terminology surrounding opioid addiction has become entirely muddled. Depending on who is doing the talking, one will hear individuals speaking of opioid dependence, physical dependence, and addiction interchangeably, when in fact these terms are absolutely not interchangeable and are quite distinct from one another.

Only adding to the confusion, the DSM-V (the 'bible' of psychiatry) refers to *opioid use disorder* when describing what is really opioid addiction. Their use of the word dependence also seems to be a little loose, depending on context. Before the DSM-V, the DSM-IV referred to *opioid dependence* when it was describing addiction. For absolute clarity, these words will be precisely defined here, so that there is no confusion about what exactly we are referring to.

Let us start with the most common phenomenon of opioid dependence. Unlike addiction, opioid dependence is *not* pathological, but rather a normal byproduct of undergoing a medical treatment that involves the use of opioids. Opioid dependence is a state of being in which the body has become accustomed to receiving opioids and now *requires*, on a cellular level, their continued administration in order to forestall withdrawal symptoms.

While this may *sound* indistinguishable from addiction, it is in fact an entirely different phenomenon and one that is, most importantly, not characterized by the appearance of cravings upon withdrawal. Opioid dependence is considered a normal and common byproduct of an extended period of opioid analgesic administration, a situation which happens frequently in longer-term hospitalized patients The neurotypical patient will manifest withdrawal symptoms upon discontinuation, but what they will not experience are the much stronger aversive hallmarks of withdrawal that are seen in addiction, which involve strong cravings in addition to experiencing the withdrawal symptoms as substantially more aversive than a neurotypical person would.

It is common medical knowledge that people who have been treated with opioids for an extended period and who then no longer require them can be tapered off of their opioid medication with little, if any, difficulty and not experience any further desire for taking the drug. This is, in fact, the reality for the vast majority of acute pain patients who are withdrawn from their medication once their painful condition has subsided. Opioid dependence is so common that every day across the country in hospitals, people are withdrawn from their pain medications with little to no fan fare. As should be clear at this point, physical opioid dependence is an entirely different phenomenon from true opioid addiction.

Opioid addiction *only* shares the physical dependence component in common with opioid dependence. That is where the commonalities end, for in the opioid addict, withdrawal is experienced as such a highly aversive state of being that cravings can often begin before the drug's half-life has even been reached. It is the nature of these cravings to be extremely powerful and to possess a compulsive element to them.

Try as they may, the addicted individual finds it impossible to distract himself from these cravings, let alone the withdrawal. As such, the withdrawal phenomenon in its totality is experienced as much *more severe* than a similar level of withdrawal would be experienced by a neurotypical individual. The nature of the cravings themselves is so total that they emanate both from the mind and the body. As the addicted individual is experiencing the physical pain from their withdrawal, their craving will be for the opioid so as to alleviate that pain. [111]

Concurrently, the psychological craving for the relief and succor that can be provided by the opioid is also extremely powerful, and it is the reason why these two forms of craving act synergistically to stack the odds against the addicted individual who is attempting to go through the withdrawal process. (see Chapter 4)

All of this having been said, readers may wonder how it is that addicts actually are able to successfully withdraw *at all*, and the answer is that though incredibly painful, withdrawal can be withstood and survived: As has been mentioned before, it is not stopping the use of opioids that is the greater challenge, it is *sustaining* that abstinence that is the seemingly unattainable holy grail for the addicted individual.

It's important to mention at this point that opioid addiction also carries with it all of the classic hallmarks of addiction such as intrusive and obsessive thoughts, loss of control over use, inability to stop using, and continued use despite adverse consequences. Furthermore, it should become clear to the reader that withdrawal from opioid dependence bears little relation to withdrawal from opioid addiction, and this is why it is so important to make the crucial distinction between the two. The thoughtful reader might be impressed by the fact that the addicted individual has a much more difficult road to traverse than does the dependent individual, so to compare the two in any way is quite unfair to the opioid addicted individual. [111,112]

A third term that has come into use relatively recently is pseudo-addiction. Pseudo-addiction is the phenomenon wherein it *appears* that a patient is exhibiting drug seeking behavior with regards to their pain medication when in reality, all the patient is doing is desperately trying to alleviate physical pain that has clearly been under-treated, thus the continued requests and appeals for analgesia.

It says something about how far we have *not* come that even legitimate patients in pain are often times viewed through the lens of "drug seeking behavior" and addiction (as a pejorative). Once again, this is entirely un-fair to the patient and places the burden and onus for pain relief on them when they are in precisely no position to obtain that pain relief without having to request it. This rapidly devolves into a double-bind/Catch-22 like no other: If you do ask, you're (potentially) damned to be labeled as drug seeking, and yet, your pain is *so bad* that you have *no choice but to ask*, all the while not knowing whether *any* relief will be attained, all because a diminishingly small handful of people have too much control over such pressing issues that some will inevitably be tempted to "play God" with your life, specifically deciding whether or not to leave you screaming in agony. [18,124]

This problem is frequently seen with patients who receive a so-called "pain pump" which is a small locked electronic box containing a reservoir of opioid drug connected directly to an external intravenous line. This box allows the pain patient to self administer doses of pain medication accord-ing to their own perceived need at the press of a button.

Unfortunately and far too often, the dosages for each individual press of the button are inadequate to relieve gradually building pain. What en-sues is an *apparently* "frantic" record of button pressing that, if interpreted incorrectly, could be viewed as drug seeking behavior when in point of fact it is the result of an insufficient dose of an opioid analgesic being adminis-tered per button press. Lest the reader misunderstand, these pain pumps are highly sophisticated electronic systems which can be programmed in such a manner so as to prevent each press of a button from automatically releas-ing opioid analgesics. They actually possess a feature which blocks the release of opioids after so many presses of the button within a prescribed period of time, predetermined by the prescribing doctor. These pain pumps often function more to spare a nurse's time than they serve to assist a pa-tient in pain with self-medicating.

Though this concept of pseudo-addiction may seem to be a relatively minor part of a larger picture or may almost seem as if we are splitting hairs, it can once again not be over emphasized that all aspects of opioid usage must be addressed if there is to be an informed discussion about this class of drugs. With that, it must be said that pseudo-addiction is not as relatively innocuous as it may seem to some readers, for there always exists the very real possibility that health care providers who *mistakenly* diagnose or suspect what (in reality) is pseudo-addiction will notate "drug seeking behavior" in the patient's medical record.

This can lead to serious repercussions for that patient's care and health outcomes, and is not to be taken lightly. Such repercussions include impairment of the healing process, as physical pain activates the body's metabolic stress systems which provoke the release of cortisol and epinephrine, both hormones that notoriously prevent the body from healing optimally, and having the label "drug seeking" placed in your permanent medical file for all posterity. *One* person's *impression* following you around whenever and wherever you may need serious medical treatment, for the rest of your life, and that (often false) impression then being acted upon by all subsequent health care professionals.

Subsequent requests for pain relief will *now* be consistently viewed through the lens of "drug seeking behavior," virtually guaranteeing that the patient will be under-medicated for pain for quite possibly the duration of their treatment, and the rest of their lives. Remember, when these notations are made, they stay in one's permanent record and follow one wherever one goes. God only knows what insurers do with this kind of sensitive information.

12

The "Why" of Opioid Addiction/ The Making of an "Addict"/ ACE's/Epigenetic changes in the brain (environment)/ Dr. Sapolsky Interview

The biggest question for most neurotypicals is *why* some people *ever* become addicted to opioids, especially considering the fact that they (the neurotypicals) are fortunate enough to be able to leave them alone when necessary. One perspective that comes to mind is that opioids produce, in certain susceptible individuals, feelings of "normality" which the person does not recognize from any other time in their lives. (138)

Most, if not all, opioid addicted individuals experience as part of this "normalization" feelings of increased energy and an increased ability to focus on tasks, something which is not seen in normal patients receiving opioids for pain.

The phenomenon in terms of the feeling of normality that many addicts report, if not that which most addicts experience, simply is not experienced by people who are exposed to opioids but do not go on to become addicted. Just reflecting on this empirical fact alone, i.e., controlling for all other variables, the sensation of normality while intoxicated appears to be a "red flag" with respect to potentially indicating who may go on to develop a true addiction to opioids. After all, opioids in general produce certain side effects, but the existential state of "feeling normal" is *not* one of them.

If people are neophytes to opioids they will experience, first and foremost, pain relief or analgesia, but then this is where the same path that they travel with those vulnerable to addiction splits because, irrespective of the fact that most pain can be controlled with opioids regardless of the individual, those individuals that do not become addicted simply do not experience a kind of event akin to a spiritual phenomenon.

It is often described by addicts as almost transcendental or metaphysical in nature. Addicts will use phrases like, "I felt like I'd come home," or, "all my life I was looking for this place." Most often the word that one hears is "normal," as in "I felt normal for the first time in my life." This sense of normality experienced by the addicted individual or potential addicted individual is so rewarding in its emotional quality as to outweigh the side effects that often accompany the use of opioids, up to and including nausea, vomiting, constipation, and even downright dysphoria.

The addicted individual who starts out as a neophyte may experience these aversive effects just as much as a person who does not go on to develop addiction, but there is something *fundamentally different* at the physiological level of the brain occurring, otherwise how else to explain the opioid addiction phenomenon and how, for that matter, it is a global phenomenon experienced in all cultures, with the clinical picture always being the same?

It is similar, for example, to the psychiatric history of schizophrenia, which was, before we had any real physiological understanding of what was going on with affected individuals and without a shred of evidence, attributed by R. D. Lang (a prominent psychiatrist in the 1960's) to bad mothering. We now know that there is an occurrence rate for schizophrenia that is identical worldwide, it is clearly not culture-bound, nor does it have any relationship to socioeconomic status, etc.

We now know that opioid addiction exists, in part, because of epigenetic changes to certain areas of the brain, as will soon be explained.

This feeling of transcendental normality is one that is nearly unexplainable, but it can be clearly explained on a physiological level. What is referred to as the "hedonic set point" is at the crux of this issue. There will always be, of populations on the "bell curve" or statistical normal distribution, a small percentage of those who are born with a biochemistry that prevents them from experiencing the simplest pleasures in life completely and fully. Instead, pleasure is experienced at a substantially diminished level. Everyday experiences for normal individuals can carry great salience *because* that salience is provided by the promise of reward: a sunrise, a fireworks display, a family gathering. [86]

There is actually a term for the aforementioned phenomenon: Reward Deficiency Syndrome. [90]

For the the addicted individual there is a very high index of suspicion, substantiated by laboratory research over the past 20 years, which clearly indicates that they require higher levels of stimulation in order to achieve what normal individuals achieve naturally and with lower, more normal levels of stimulation. In part this explains how, even though there is no such thing as an addictive personality, there are sets of *behaviors* that one can observe in susceptible individuals prodromally that would indicate that those individuals are at a higher risk for addiction. These behaviors have in common that they involve activities that *tend* not to attract neurotypicals.

For potential addicts, expressed behaviors that *are* satisfying *tend* to be risky activities, and will often be taken to an extreme. Some examples would be bungee jumpers, base jumpers, or people involved in extreme sports. Essentially, they desire ever greater "peak experiences." The outer limits of such activities would for most neurotypical people be experienced as aversive, if not downright terrifying. [88]

There are clear indices that can be observed empirically with research that has been conducted over the last two decades, research that is clinical, published and peer reviewed, which indicates that addiction, like any other mental illness, is partially the result of a dysfunction within the brain. How is an addicted individual's brain different from a neurotypical's brain? As before, the answer lies partially in the fact that the addicted individual's brain has a deficit in the ability to *fully* experience any given positive stimulus. It will not produce for the addicted individual the same level of pleasure that it will in a neurotypical individual's brain, given the same positive stimulus.

Here, one can see the ontological basis of addiction for a vulnerable individual who finally experiences a level of pleasure that they have never experienced before in their lives. This may be difficult for neurotypical individuals to conceive of, but after the point of first use, when the vulnerable individual experiences a normally pleasant stimulus, it will pale even further in comparison to before, to the point where it may feel utterly vacuous. This is because before they ever became addicted, these individuals' experiences of positive stimuli did not produce normal levels of pleasure. The now often-mentioned sunrise that might thrill a neurotypical individual would be experienced by an addicted individual at a greatly diminished level such that the person may observe it as a nebulously pleasant natural phenomenon and then ask themselves, "what's the big deal?" or "what's next?" [88]

The most comprehensive concept that needs to be understood, repetitive analogies set aside, is an absolutely holistic analogy appropriate to further understand this concept. If one can imagine two children being born, one neurotypical and the other not, as they grow into young children, adolescents and then adults, the neurotypical individual, simply by dint of enjoying a certain level of reward that a stimulus appropriately provides, perceives a certain reality and world-view that allows them to see life through a proverbial set of rose colored glasses much like other neurotypical's do; the unfortunate vulnerable individual, from birth to adulthood, tends to be more prone to melancholy and a "the glass is half empty" natural bent towards pessimism, and, most importantly, they don't enjoy the same level of reward for the same stimulus that produces that reward for the majority population. [88]

American society is replete with more guns than citizens, yet for some reason, our society believes that a *weapon of war* (such as an AR-15) should be the birthright of every citizen/person to own, no questions asked. It seems odd because the firearm, which though it can be used for suicide, can also be (and is often) used offensively, while chemical substances, which simply effect the body of the individual ingesting them and no one else, are considered the bane of our current culture. This is a uniquely American paradox considering how much emphasis our fellow citizens place on individuality and the right for every person to determine their own fate.

As has been mentioned at the beginning of this book, researchers have discovered that certain strains of lab rats are *much* more prone to addiction-like behavior than are others. [5] Strains of animal species are roughly equivalent to human consanguineous families; the human corollary of this is that addiction tends to run in families. Why would humans be much different? [126]

Why some people *continue* to use opioids no matter the consequences (the definition of addiction) is a question that has only recently begun to receive answers, and one of the main answers appears to lay in the newer science of epigenetics. Epigenetics is the study of changes in gene activity and expression that can be heritable. The key point to remember is that while some genes may be silenced and others expressed, there is *no change* whatsoever in the fundamental DNA template.

What happens in the addicted individual's brain is that with regular opioid use, certain genes get turned on, while others get turned off. Once these changes in genetic expression occur, they can be so long lasting as to be effectively irreversible. The fact that these irreversible changes happen in an addicted individual's brain is something that is believed to be genetically determined, and expressed through contact with the environment, i.e. opioids. These changes occur in areas of the brain that are crucially involved in motivation, planning, and executive functioning. [85]

The other, uniquely human element to the reason why some people ever use opioids to begin with goes back to another topic mentioned at the beginning of this book, the issue of Adverse Childhood Experiences (ACEs). The ACE's study is the first of its kind to discover a direct correlation between ACEs experienced by individuals and a subsequent, dose-related increase in individual mortality and morbidity from all causes, and because of its' sheer statistical power, the conclusions are undeniable: The more adversity a child experiences, the worse their health outcomes are *decades later*. [9]

This last point cannot be overemphasized: even though children in toxic environments usually escape those environments in young adulthood, the damage caused by the toxic stress has already been established for a lifetime. And that damage takes the form of dramatically elevated rates of morbidity and mortality from nearly all causes, e.g. cardiovascular, metabolic, psychiatric, etc., etc. [7,103,104]

Perhaps the most astonishing finding for the purposes of this book is that a child who has had "only" four aces (out of a possible grand total of ten) is **ten** times more likely to become an injection drug user, **seven** times as likely to become alcoholic, and **twelve** times more likely to attempt suicide. [9,10]

These are truly astonishing numbers and yet when they were first published, up until today, there has been *no national dialogue* about how morbidity and mortality are so strongly "selected for" in childhood. True, academia continues this important work to this day, but there has been *zero* open acknowledgement of these findings in the media. Perhaps Americans are not yet ready to hear the arguably most important finding of the 21st century, namely that pedagogy matters, and it matters much more than had ever previously been realized or suspected.

America, it can be said, is the most individualistic society in the West, and this may help explain why the ACE Study findings went over like a lead balloon with the general public – In a country where home schooling is a legal option for those who wish to "drop out" of society, it's hard to imagine people being thrilled about being "told how to raise (their) children," especially when that information comes from already distrusted academic institutions of higher learning.

Taking a page from the anti-vaccination crowd of parents who refuse to get their children vaccinated for whatever reason, it appears that society-at-large is willfully ignoring the most crucial evidence from these undeniable (and since reproduced) results, namely that _a child's environment has a much more powerful influence on the course of the rest of their lives than had ever been realized, potentially more powerful than any other factor._

"The current studies demonstrate that across reward classes, early-life adversity causes robust and consistent deficits in the hedonic processing of rewards." [94]

"It is not the purview of this book to discuss the ACEs Study at length, however, there are a number of online resources to guide readers further interested in this subject that can easily be found via a simple Google search."

"Drug abuse (DA) is an etiologically complex syndrome strongly influenced by a diverse set of genetic risk factors reflecting a specific liability to DA, by a vulnerability to other externalizing disorders, and by a range of environmental factors reflecting marital instability, as well as psychopathology and criminal behavior in the adoptive home. *Adverse environmental effects on DA are more pathogenic in individuals with high levels of genetic risk.*" [87] [ed. note: *emphasis added*]

The above quote comes from another statistical powerhouse of a study (like the ACEs study,) Genetic and Familial Environmental Influences on the Risk for Drug Abuse: A National Swedish Adoption Study. Again, as we saw with the ACEs study, the reason why this study's conclusions are so solid is because the authors looked at more than *18,000* adopted children born between 1950 and 1993 *longitudinally* with respect to a measure they call Drug Abuse (DA.) This study was published in 2012, and for all of its wordiness, its conclusion is simple enough: "Drug Abuse" runs in biological relatives, even if a child is adopted out early from a biological parental environment of drug abuse. [87]

Another important conclusion has been arrived at by this study: Genetics may be crucial for predisposition (i.e. vulnerability,) but environment has a tremendous impact on genetics. Said another way, vulnerability *must meet with* adversity and exposure to produce a person who abuses drugs.

Interestingly, this study also indirectly confirms the ACE Study conclusions regarding childhood traumata and later, adult morbidity and mortality.

"Finally, we analyzed these predictor variables on the scale of raw probabilities without and with an interaction between the genetic and environmental risk scores... The interaction was significant, showing that the impact of an adverse environment on risk for DA was substantially greater in those with a high vs low genetic liability to DA." [87]

"Fifth, we found evidence for gene-environment interaction in the etiology of DA. Adopted children at high genetic risk were more sensitive to the pathogenic effects of adverse family environments than those at low genetic risk. In other words, genetic effects on DA were less potent in low-risk than in high-risk environments. These results are consistent with prior twin studies suggesting that genetic influences on psychoactive substance use in adolescence are enhanced in high-risk environments characterized by low parental monitoring, easy substance availability, and the presence of substance-using friends, as well as consistent with molecular genetic studies showing that *risk variants may interact positively with familial environmental adversity in the prediction of DA.*" [87] [ed. note: *emphasis added*]

"a range of environmental features of the adoptive family predicted risk for DA in adopted children. *Unlike prior studies in intact families, the causal chain between these risk factors and DA is not confounded by genetic relationships between family members. These diverse risk factors include disruption of the marital and parent-child bonds through death or divorce, alcohol problems in the adoptive parents or siblings, and criminal behavior and medical hospitalization in the adoptive parents.*" [87] [ed. note: *emphasis added*]

Work on this book has brought the author in contact with Dr. Robert Sapolsky, currently a professor of biology, and professor of neurology and neurological sciences and, by courtesy, neurosurgery, at Stanford University. He was kind enough to answer several very specific questions regarding ACEs, opioid addiction, and resilience to adversity, [11]

Q: When considering the CDC's original Adverse Childhood Experience's study, what relative role do ACE's have, particularly as the number of adverse events increase, on the development of opioid addiction in vulnerable individuals?

A: "I suspect there are a bunch of paths from lots of ACEs to adult addiction – for example, the fact that a lot of ACEs effects frontal cortical development in a way that make people very steep temporal discounters – why wait for a good reward tomorrow when you can have an unhealthy one now? For my money, I think the biggest effects of ACEs is via stress effects on development of the dopamine system

– predisposing individuals towards depression and anxiety (and with the resulting increased odds of falling into self-medicating), and *making for a system that is, in general, less responsive to typical rewards.*" [ed. note: *emphasis added*]

Q: Is the nature of the vulnerability-factor with addicts so great that said individuals, if exposed to the right environment, will become addicts irrespective of their psychological histories?

A: "It's probably something akin to the trauma literature, where there are people whose biological vulnerability is so high that they are flattened by the smallest of challenges, and people whose biological resilience is so great that they come out of the Holocaust relatively psychologically intact."

Q: With reference to the aforementioned ACE's, what mediating role do you feel glucocorticoids (and also CRF) have with respect to the resultant increased morbidity and mortality, irrespective of whether or not the affected individual goes on to opioid addiction or not?

A: "A tremendous role, particularly in terms of *the effects of glucocorticoids (and CRF) on the developing brain.*" [ed. note: *emphasis added*]

As can be clearly seen from Dr. Sapolsky's answers to my questions, stress plays an enormous role in raising the vulnerability of the young, developing brain to addiction, and this goes a long way toward explaining why early ACEs can be so destructive throughout a persons entire life-span. [21]

The way that stress mediates addiction vulnerability is via, as Dr. Sapolsky had indicated earlier,

"Physiological responses (are) manifested through the two major stress pathways, namely *corticotropin releasing factor (CRF)* released from the paraventricular nucleus (PVN) of the hypothalamus, *which stimulates adrenocorticotropin hormone from the anterior pituitary, which subsequently stimulates the secretion of cortisol* (a glucocorticoid) from the adrenal glands, and the auto-nomic nervous system, which is coordinated via the sympathoad-renal medulary (SAM) systems." [21] [ed. note: *emphases added*]

One of the main stress hormones that is secreted during stressful challenge is cortisol, and cortisol is a glucocorticoid hormone (GH,) *the* glucocorti-coid hormone, which is secreted by the adrenal glands in response to cor-ticosteroid releasing factor (CRF) secreted by the pituitary gland in the brain. The take-away from this is that GHs increase a person's risk for developing an addictive disorder because they can have adverse effects on the *developing brain*, effects that include impairing proper development of the frontal cortex.

"Neurobiological evidence shows that with increasing levels of stress, there is a decrease in prefrontal functioning and increased limbic-striatal level responding, which perpetuates low behavioral and cognitive control. Thus, *the motivational brain pathways are key targets of brain stress chem-icals* and provide an important potential mechanism by which stress affects addiction vulnerability." [21] [ed. note: *emphasis added*]

To make matters worse, GHs *sensitize* certain critical areas of the brain to the effects of potentially addictive drugs.

"In conclusion, our results indicate that glucocorticoids, via GRs (glu-cocorticoid receptors,) facilitate dopamine-dependent behavioral effects of morphine, probably by modifying dopamine release." [98]

"Early-life stress and prolonged and repeated stress also adversely af-fect development of the prefrontal cortex (PFC,) a region that is highly dependent on environmental experiences for maturation. The PFC, and particularly the right PFC, plays an important role both in activating the hypothalamic-pituitary-adrenal (HPA) axis and autonomic responses to stress and in regulating these responses." [21]

The reason why the pre-frontal cortex (PFC) can play such a tremen-dous role in someone's life is because the PFC is what allows us to control volitional behaviors, or as Dr. Sapolsky would say, the PFC "makes you do the harder thing when that is the right thing to do." [106] Stress can impair proper development of the pre-frontal and frontal cortex, and this can be so detrimental at such a young age precisely because the frontal cortex is the very last part of the human brain to mature, and it is highly dependent on environmental experiences for maturation. [106]

The range of potential stressors is quite broad, however they all have an element of *unpredictability* to them.

"the dose-dependent effects of cumulative stressors on risk for addiction existed for both genders and for Caucasian, African-American, and Hispanic race/ethnic groups. The types of adverse events significantly associated with addiction vulnerability were parental divorce or conflict, abandonment, forced to live apart from parents, loss of child by death or removal, unfaithfulness of significant other, loss of home to natural disaster, death of a close one, emotional abuse or neglect, sexual abuse, rape, physical abuse by parent, caretaker, family member, spouse, or significant other, victim of gun shooting or other violent acts, and observing violent victimization." [21]

These all represent highly stressful and emotionally distressing events, which are typically uncontrollable and unpredictable in nature.

To sum up the main factors involved in the risk for addiction, we have come around full-circle to the three usual suspects.

"...three types of vulnerability factors: (1) developmental/individual-level factors such as frontal executive function development, negative emotionality, behavioral/self-control, impulsivity, or risk taking, and altered initial sensitivity to rewarding effects of drugs; (2) stress-related vulnerability factors such as early adverse life events, trauma and child maltreatment experiences, prolonged and chronic stress experiences; and (3) genetic influences and family history of psychopathology and addiction, which have not been discussed here but have significant interactive effects on addiction risk and in emotion and stress markers." [21]

13

FALLING DOWN THE RABBIT HOLE-FAILED TREATMENT MODALITIES

ULTRA RAPID DETOXIFICATION

Rapid detoxification, sometimes known as Ultra Rapid Detoxification or UROD, is a relatively new player on the scene of addiction treatment. For those readers unfamiliar with UROD, a brief synopsis follows. The opioid addicted individual is admitted to a hospital facility or surgery center and under the supervision of anesthesiologists and other physicians, the patient is placed under general anesthesia. It is during this time of unconsciousness that the patient is then given opioid antagonists, most commonly naltrexone, which serves to replace the opioids that are attached to the receptors in the brain with the naltrexone itself. As naltrexone is known as a full opioid antagonist, a very severe form of withdrawal is induced in the anesthetized patient, the *idea* being that withdrawal could be accomplished during the entire time that the patient is under anesthesia so that they do not experience the physical symptoms of withdrawal and once they are awakened from the unconscious state, they are no longer physically opioid dependent.

If it ended there, this would be the ideal treatment for opioid addiction, however, in reality, there are a tremendous number of physiological aftereffects which reveal that this process is anything but painless and usually results, among other things, in a disastrous relapse.

The reason why relapses are so common after UROD are two fold. First, though the person is (usually) no longer physically addicted to opioids, because of the rapid onset of Post Acute Withdrawal Syndrome or PAWS which occurs after UROD is completed (this is written about at length in Chapter 4), the patient begins to experience intense cravings for opioids to alleviate the complete anhedonia, or utter and total inability to feel or experience pleasure, that is present.

Anhedonia is such a potent contributor to relapse because the ability to experience any kind of pleasure is such an integral part of what makes us feel human, such that when one is in an anhedonic state one literally feels utterly and entirely disconnected from the world around them, rendering one relegated to living in a world in which they are breathing, but not alive.

Unfortunately, severe anhedonia is only one of many potential after effects of UROD. Other effects can include severe insomnia such that the patient may experience a total inability to sleep, and this total lack of sleep can last for weeks which subsequently can give way to months of fractured sleep, fractured sleep simply meaning that the patient awakens many times during the night, never quite reaching the full benefit of a healthy sleep cycle.

Because a sleep cycle requires a minimum of 90 minutes to achieve, fractured sleep will render the patient feeling as though they haven't slept at all. These two factors alone are a tremendous setup for relapse, but they are the are not the only two factors at play for the UROD patient.

Since each UROD provider uses essentially their own protocol, patients can sometimes awaken and still be in withdrawal. UROD can prove to be immediately disastrous in such a situation and this scenario has been documented to have happened. Furthermore, there have been documented fatalities as a result of the anesthesia or other failures in the providers established protocol.

Most UROD practitioners include in their protocol administration of naltrexone tablets daily post-UROD to the freshly withdrawn patient in order to safeguard against potential overdose should the patient be unable to withstand the intense cravings and psychic pain that are more the rule than the exception with this form of treatment. Some providers have even taken to administering long lasting intramuscular injections of naltrexone to promote patient compliance, and patient compliance is precisely the second part of why UROD does not work in the long term. [84]

Patients may initially comply with their naltrexone prescription orders, however, this compliance lasts at best for two to three weeks until the patient makes the connection that taking the naltrexone tablet *intensifies* their anhedonia. Naltrexone has this effect because it does not discriminate in its blockade of opioid action between exogenous and endogenous opioids. Endogenous opioids, most commonly referred to as endorphins, are our body's own natural morphine. We experience rushes of them when we go for a good jog, when we enjoy a nice slice of chocolate cake or when we experience a beautiful sunrise or when we are with someone we love deeply. The hedonic, or reward blockade, is so total and complete that the patient eventually stops taking the naltrexone so that they can feel *anything* at all. And who can blame them?

It is important to note that this anhedonic effect of naltrexone is only experienced by former opioid addicts, but it is not experienced by alcoholic patients who take naltrexone to reduce their drinking.

It is an admittedly very seductive notion that for some money and a short stint in the hospital one can bypass all of the aversive qualities of withdrawal without being conscious, however, real experience has shown that this is not possible for the vast majority of addicted individuals, irrespective of how committed or eager they are to shed themselves of their addiction.

This brings us to why UROD can be so dangerous to opioid addicts who wish to rid themselves of their addiction. In point of fact, if UROD is properly done, the patient will no longer be *physically* addicted to opioids, and therein lies the problem; overnight, they have gone from being highly tolerant of opioids to having zero tolerance. Were the naltrexone actually a feasible part of the protocol, relapse would not be so dangerous, however, it is precisely because the compliance with naltrexone is so poor that patients are rendered incredibly susceptible and vulnerable to an overdose if relapse occurs. [83]

For example, if before they underwent UROD they were using 50 mg.

of heroin a day and then after undergoing treatment they attempt to use that same dosage during a relapse, that could very well prove lethal, since as far as the body is concerned, the tolerance that once existed for the patient ended with the conclusion of the UROD. [80,81,82]

FAITH BASED APPROACH

Another horrible idea when it comes to helping opioid addicted individuals is in the form of what is known as faith based treatment. A simple Google search will produce countless results for these sorts of facilities. As their names imply, this form of treatment relies upon faith in a supernatural being, in western societies usually a Christian god, to heal afflicted individuals of their addiction, which is often times viewed and presented to the addicted individual as being the result of a fundamentally spiritual problem, i.e. that one is possessed by evil forces or that one is estranged from God, or that one is rebelling against their faith and that the addiction is a manifestation of that rebellion, etc.

To understand that this type of treatment cannot work, all one has to do is look at the recurring headlines of children who have died because their parents have refused them medical care on the premise that God, according to the holy scriptures, will heal their children by faith alone. Clearly, if faith doesn't work for cancer or a simple infection, why would it work for an entrenched drug addiction?

A less discussed problem with faith based treatment is the mentally cruel effect it can have upon individuals availing themselves of such treatment, specifically that this treatment modality is fundamentally cruel to a persons inner spiritual life because it implicitly places the onus for getting better or staying off of drugs on one's perceived level of spiritual "commitment," leaving him or her not only just as sick as they were before, but now also psychically injured as they are left feeling alienated and judged from the very faith they sought help from. Faith is not medical care. It can serve as a spiritual balm or at best as an adjunctive therapy, but on it's own, it is as effective as a placebo. If it were efficacious, we would have no need for hospitals, pharmacies or the scientific community producing cutting edge research.

COLD TURKEY ABSTINENCE

Abstinence in general is an approach to recovering from opioid addiction that has largely been proven to not only be ineffective, but actually in fact quite dangerous. For the sake of readers to whom it may not seem obvious, here are some simple reasons why. Cold Turkey withdrawal from opioids, particularly short acting opioids like heroin, morphine, oxycodone, etc., is simply, but not easily, accomplished. In this respect, Mark Twain comes to mind when he spoke of quitting tobacco, saying *"Giving up **smoking** is the easiest thing in the world. I know because I've done it thousands of times."*

And just like Mark Twain, with opioid addicted individuals, *quitting* opioids is not the actual fundamental difficulty. It is in *staying off* of opioids over the long term that abstinence proves itself to be as elusive as the holy grail. For arguments sake, even for those addicted individuals who manage to string together a significant amount of opioid-free time, even stretching into years, there is a not insignificant and ever present danger of relapse due to the unremittingly chronic nature of true opioid addiction. It is within relapsing that opioid addiction can be particularly lethal since, by definition, the person relapsing, having lost all the tolerance they once had, is most vulnerable to an overdose.

Cold Turkey abstinence is, by definition, a form of abstinence that is achieved through sheer grit and determination or incarceration, but completely in the absence of any kind of external medical support. It should not come as a surprise then that people who choose this route tend to relapse rather quickly since they experience severe PAWS as soon as their acute withdrawal is over. The reality with PAWS is that even under the best of circumstances, it can dissipate into the ether only to return with a vengeance at a time of its own choosing so that it is impossible for the addicted individual or anyone to predict. On the deepest level, what this is most likely about are the fundamental and permanent brain changes that are wrought by the opioids on the brain's limbic system, also known as our reward system, via epigenetic modifications to the brain's cells.(see Chapter 12)

It is hypothesized that as with cocaine addiction, these changes are in the form of what are known as epigenetic changes to the actual DNA within the brains neurons. Epigenetics is a term used to describe heritable physical changes that do not involve alterations in the DNA sequence, but rather changes in a gene's activity and expression. Crucial to this definition is that these effects may result from normal development processes or external environmental factors. The fascinating thing about epigenetics is that the physical changes observed can potentially be passed on to subsequent generations, although this has still not been established with any degree of absolute certainty.

12 STEP PROGRAMS

Since your brick-and-mortar 12 step programs operate under the simple principle of total and absolute abstinence, there is little more that can be said for these programs since they are asking their opioid addicted supplicants to subscribe to the philosophy that abstaining "one day at a time" is going to produce therapeutic success over the long term, all empirical evidence to the contrary.

For readers unfamiliar with the 12 step philosophy, it is in essence a philosophy where the afflicted individual assumes an *absolute responsibility for their affliction* that to some seems excessive considering what is *now* known about the etiology of addiction, opioid addiction in particular. As such, a good part of 12 step program work is involved in admitting ones own failures and in making amends to people whom one may have wronged or injured.

As Dr. Gabor Mate has so brilliantly pointed out, an enormous problem with this lies precisely in the fact that so many opioid addicted individuals are *themselves* often disproportionately victims of some form or another of abuse, that to ask such individuals to assume total responsibility for their own injuries is akin to blaming the victim for their aggressor's sins. What needs to always be kept in mind is that precisely because of the frequently tragic histories of opioid addicts, this treatment modality *can* actually end up making an addicted individual's situation *worse*.

A huge confounding factor in 12-step programs is the tremendous camaraderie that usually attends these meetings. An emotional intimacy develops and is shared with a large group of people and it can easily mask some deeper, more subconscious difficulties with one's recovery. Specifically, by providing a wide social network the 12 step message is reinforced but the individual's biological processes for relapse remain on track and unimpeded, because ultimately, opioid addiction is not a social disease, it is biological in nature and as such requires a medical solution. [8,42]

In all fairness, it would be a disservice to discount the social and emotional benefit that millions of people derive from attending 12 step organizations and activities, just as it would be unfair to those opioid addicted individuals to discount the very real biological processes that are taking place in their brains, whether they attend meetings or not.

MISCELLANEOUS "LUXURY" REHAB CENTERS

Perhaps the most egregious violations of medical ethics occur in for-profit rehabilitation facilities, particularly the ones that cater to very high end, wealthy clientèle that can afford to either pay out-of-pocket or with generous insurance company reimbursements upwards of 100K a month for what amount to little more than luxury getaways that focus on all sorts of nebulous mind-body "holistic" treatment modalities that ostensibly "cure" their guests of all of their unwanted addictions. While it cannot be argued that a month of pampering and one-on-one attention *won't* do a body good, the same biological imperatives that attend pure abstinence also apply to this treatment protocol.

Once one has left the confines of the oceanside retreat with daily massages, world class cuisine and one-on-one daily therapy as well as group therapy treatments, one is sent back to his or her traditional environs with all of the same stressors and temptations, with the sole admonition to attend 12 step meetings and to "call if you need us." That these forms of rehabilitation don't work in the long term is clearly attested to by the countless celebrities that use them as revolving doors in a misguided attempt to obtain long-term recovery. [78]

In a closing statement here, it must be stated for the record that "celebrity doctors" like Dr. "Drew" Pinsky, M.D. (and his ilk, like "Dr. Phil", Ph.D.) are doing *incalculable damage* to the opioid-addicted population that is still desperately looking for answers and effective treatment. If you have a medical degree, or a doctorate of psychology, respectively, you have no business steering an opioid addicted individual into abstinence-based treatment, *and then making it seem like that is their only realistic choice for treatment*: After all, **you know better**. If you *really don't*, most patients would be very discomforted to be made aware of that. Again, this isn't "cutting-edge" science here, something that has only been known for a decade or two. We have known about the realities of opioid addiction for *generations*.

In the face of what has been known for *over 100 years* about the "incurability" of true opioid addiction, this can only leave the impression that the staggering post-treatment death rate for (abstinent) opioid addicts is, in some way or another, the *only* socially acceptable answer to this problem, or, to use the (somewhat infamous) words of 12 Step programs, "Some of us have to die, so that others may live."

That a noted physician *and* psychologist would, in 2020, still endorse *abstinence only* as a valid recovery tool from opioid addiction is, in actuality, the pinnacle of immorality itself. The sheer persistence of abstinence only *mythology* in precisely those circles that should know far better only serves to confirm the dominant narrative of the hated and feared junkie as a societal bogeyman, entirely in spite of the *fact* that the conclusion of that narrative is almost always death or further institutionalization.

14

DEATH AFTER FAILED ABSTINENCE

We would be irresponsible to not recognize that having to suffer the physical and psychological experiences of withdrawal are immeasurably more difficult to cope with in a penal institution than they are in the privacy of ones own home, or at a medical facility. Let us make no mistake nor underestimate the explosiveness of this issue: This is a *human rights issue* where, in some jurisdictions, the State feels itself impervious to either scrutiny or prosecution for essentially exacting "cruel and unusual punishment" that could be completely avoided with the simple administration of methadone and other necessary medications. [77]

The sum total amount of payouts to families of victims who have *died* from withdrawal while incarcerated is unknowable, so it can only be deduced that the practice of "cruelly and unusually" punishing an inmate suffering from addiction, before a trial and conviction ever take take place, is more jurisprudentially satisfying than administering lifesaving medications that cost pennies on the dollar. Society's disdain for those that suffer from addiction serves as an unspoken endorsement for this punitive approach, and therein lies the ultimate conundrum. [51,52]

As is discussed in more detail in Chapter 18, it is imperative that the MMT patient avoid incarceration at all costs. This is, when one thinks it through, rather simple to accomplish. Avoid even simple unpaid parking tickets, as they have cost at least one person his life. [73,74] Avoid any and all activities which could even be construed as illegal. By the time you are in a holding cell, it is already too late for effective redress.

Clearly, the crimes committed against humanity during WWII that started with the dehumanization of entire groups of people could only have happened because a majority of people chose to look the other way or chose not to care. In organizations that already have a core of authoritarianism, this kind of passive acquiescence to authority is simply and shrewdly taken by the powers-that-be as *complicity*. Such organizations, for example, would naturally include the necessary institutions of society such as local and state police and the federal justice system, which all share in common a top-down hierarchy of "justice." It is hardly imaginable that most citizens would be comfortable with the knowledge of having been complicit in an extrajudicial execution. [108]

The problem with this kind of "justice" that is being delivered to addicted individuals is that when we take the actual situation of forced withdrawal and compare it to the simple laws of the land, it would be hard to argue that these jailhouse and/or prison deaths are not the essential equivalent of extrajudicial torture and summary execution, with the perpetrators feeling entirely justified and the dead having neither recourse nor remedy. [75,108] One can only guess that the administrators of this perversion of justice are left with a certain degree of satisfaction at having removed "one more" member of an element that is so ubiquitously unwanted and ostracized from every strata of society, often including their own families. [77]

This brings one to ponder the question of whether the current deafening silence by the public regarding these extrajudicial crimes is active, passive, or more a result of the fact that these incidents are so rarely publicized, and when they *are* reported they are often given the blurb treatment, with the timbre of articles smacking of the attitude that "they had it coming," or that their deaths were the end result of fate or (perhaps cruelest of all) entirely chosen of free will by the decedent. Opioid addiction and it's sequelae are, unfortunately, nearly universally considered an active choice. Jailhouse-withdrawal deaths happen and have happened more frequently than the general public would expect, and it can safely be said that every one of them was *avoidable*. [75]

There are a number of reasons that jail administrators advance as to why they do not as a matter of routine administer any kind of controlled substances to inmates, irrespective of whether the controlled substance has been legitimately prescribed and, in the case of some controlled substances, is literally necessary for the continued sustenance of life. [76] One can only suspect that the most typical reason follows the conventional wisdom that since an addicted individual is, in the public's mind, nothing but a self-circulating machine of hedonistic self-indulgence, a good way to "teach them a lesson" is to let them experience pain, not understanding the fact that *no amount* of punishment, pain, torture or even threat of death will ultimately stop an affected individual that is truly addicted from using opioids again.

Volition plays no role in an opioid addicted individual, therefore punishment is an absurd concept, considering that you are punishing them for a condition that they themselves don't want to have in the first place. The point here is that the punishment idea is what is behind every ineffective *non-evidence-based* treatment modality from therapeutic communities to the old narcotics farm in Lexington Kentucky, up to and including today's contemporary, expensive, and "in vogue" treatment facilities like "Passages Malibu." (see Chapter 13)

The second, more unconscious and archetypal reason that has spread throughout society is that drug addicts are believed to be disproportionately responsible for levels of criminality and social problems that are actually out of proportion to their numbers, and it is because of the persistence of this belief that opioid addicted individuals and injection drug users are considered to be the ultimate in lawlessness. These stereotypes appeal to society's most primal, basest fears. Joe Q. Public tenaciously holds onto these negative and factually baseless attitudes even though most have never encountered an actual opioid addicted individual *per se*.

A simple analogy is demonstrated by the fact that the term "skid row" has fallen out of use when speaking of alcoholism, *because* there is a general public awareness and a growing acknowledgment that alcoholism is, in point of fact, a disease that is quite amenable to treatment, with a diminishingly small number of sufferers that are treatment resistant.

In June 2015, 32-year-old David Stojcevski, a Detroit man enrolled in a medication-assisted treatment (MAT) program, died while serving a 30-day sentence for careless driving. David underwent at least five violations of the Geneva Conventions on basic human rights (to which the United States was one of the first signatories.) In court in Macomb, Michigan, he had been ordered to pay a fine of $655 for a simple driving infraction, a sum that he was not able to come up with, and thus chose a 30 day period of incarceration to settle his debt to society. Upon entering the jail, he notified the intake officers that he was a methadone maintenance patient and that he also had a prescription for a benzodiazepine for an anxiety disorder he suffered from. [73,108,110]

Though these are both controlled substances he was well *within his rights* to receive, his first day of incarceration disabused him of that notion, as he was given neither his prescribed methadone nor his anti-anxiety medication. As the hours ticked into days, Mr. Stojcevski progressively became, at an accelerating pace, more debilitated and ill to the point where by day 17 he died in his cell, naked on the floor, 50 lbs lighter than when he was admitted due to uncontrolled vomiting and diarrhea brought on by forced withdrawal, and status epilepticus brought on by cold-turkey withdrawal of benzodiazepines, without having had any medical intervention which could have *easily* prevented his death, that being the administration of his prescribed medications. The reader may ask how and why this happened to an American citizen. This question is one that leads us in the right direction, however, the answers that have been provided are less than satisfying and leave much to be desired. [72-77,108,110]

The first place that this completely understandable and normal question should lead us to is a good first clue, namely the question of, "What role and responsibility does the media have with respect to the greatest good for the greatest number of citizens that rely simply on what the media apparatus is putting out there?" As civilians, we can not act upon injustices that we are not even aware of, and this informative role is the job of our collective news media. [79]

Until media reporting *truly* becomes more egalitarian, we will continue to be utterly unaware of what is going on around the corner in our community's local jail. Patrick Moynahan famously stated that, "all politics is local". This statement has only become more true with the passing of time, due to the consolidation of our traditional media outlets/providers to literally a handful of families who dynastically own and run most of the traditional media that we rely on for information. [51,52,69,70]

15

"KROKODIL" AND OTHER STREET SUBSTITUTES OR, IF EVER THERE WAS A REASON TO QUIT...

If ever there was hardcore proof that *no amount* of punishment can deter an opioid addict, we need look no further than the phenomenon of 'Krokodil' that has overtaken the Russian Republic (federation).

For those readers not yet familiar with this nightmare of a drug, it is almost exclusively produced in the Russian Federation and former member states of the Soviet Union. The reason for this is that Russia is the only major country in the world that has *outlawed* MAT and harm reduction techniques like needle-exchanges. The situation for opioid addicted individuals there is currently *so bad* that these must be referred to as *basic human rights violations*, for Russia is willfully ignoring the juggernaut-mass of evidence-based data indicating the success of MAT and harm-reduction. Their ostensible reason is that they "don't want to substitute one drug for another," among other more ridiculous reasons... sound familiar?

So now, the Russian Federation has two million desperate opioid addicts who cannot always easily obtain heroin or other substitutes, not to mention an unacceptable rate of new HIV infections every year. (136) If necessity is the mother of invention, then Krokodil is the invention from the bowels of hell. Krokodil is a very crudely "cooked" form of desomorphine which is easily made from tablets containing codeine. The drawback is that the process is so dirty and loaded with contaminants that users end up dramatically poisoning themselves on an installment plan, so to speak.

In addition, because desomorphine is so short-acting (2-3 hours,) even addicted individuals who know chemistry and could "clean up" their product have little time before the advent of intense withdrawal symptoms...and so it goes in a vicious cycle.

The toxic brew that is Krokodil is so poisonous that people's skin becomes scaly and leathery (thus, the name "Crocodile",) an effect which appears essentially irreversible. Users bodies become covered in abscesses and pustules, and not infrequently, they begin to lose flesh from areas of their bodies. Survival of these walking dead is estimated to be <5 years from starting Krokodil use. [136,137]

If anything were an incentive to quit, I would think it would be the dreadful aforementioned effects of Krokodil, and yet, this is not what is being seen in Russia. We are only seeing a displacement of sources for codeine containing headache tablets, but not a reduction in people making Krokodil. This comes as no surprise to the author, but it may surprise some neurotypicals into realizing that there are *no consequences bad enough that will make opioid addicts stay abstinent*, they just do not exist. The fact that people don't quit Krokodil as much as they *die from it* is litmus-test proof that even fear of immanent death is not enough to stop opioid addicts.

There is another human side to this story, and it has everything to do with massive ethical violations on the part of Russian healthcare personnel. As Krokodil first flooded the Russian opioid scene, Russian hospitals and doctors would release filmed footage of some of these desperate souls, often times with no clothes on whatsoever, and I highly suspect that the patients were not engaged in informed consent with respect to their filming. I have seen a number of these films on the internet and they are shocking in how they display physicians and nurses treating these dying people like freak-show objects. In one video, a physician can be seen rhythmically tapping a pencil on the entirely bare forearm bone of a naked patient as if she were a xylophone.

There is little that the West can do about these kinds of human rights abuses in Russia, but one suggestion for people who want to make a difference is to contact your local Amnesty International office to ask how you can help. They're never at a surplus for "foot-soldiers," and they appreciate the help that volunteers bring.

16

A TALE OF TWO CLINICS

What follows is a comparison between two different Methadone Maintenance Treatment (MMT) facilities in America today, one located in Chicago, Illinois, and the other in Detroit, MI. [138] The differences between these clinics are illustrative of the spectral differences present between all clinics. As it now stands, each methadone clinic in the United States is really an island unto itself.

What this effectively means is that because federal guidelines stipulate that methadone is to be dispensed only from specialized clinics, there is already an inherent problem with those guidelines in that they intentionally and entirely remove the delivery of MMT services from the general healthcare system, rendering the services they deliver up to the whims, preferences and prejudices of each individual owner/operator. This can foreseeably result in vastly different experiences and outcomes that are determined entirely by the geographic location one is either lucky or unlucky enough to find oneself in. That this current state of affairs exists, and is grossly unfair, will be made eminently clear by the end of this section.

In Chicago, John opened the door to a large MMT clinic with an exceedingly pleasant décor that contained a children's play area. As John looked around, he could not help but be impressed by how clean, bright and welcoming the facility appeared. As he made himself comfortable in the well appointed waiting room that was outfitted with comfortable chairs and plenty of current reading materials, he awaited his prescheduled appointment time. After his name was called by a nurse, he walked to the front desk and made a mental note of the demeanor of the staff behind the desk. It was exceedingly congenial and friendly, indistinguishable from the medical professionals he encountered when he visited his primary care physician or dentist's office.

As John made his way into the dosing area, he was immediately struck by the lack of any kind of physical barrier between patients and the nurses who dispensed the methadone. He was engaged by the nurse in common, friendly banter about the weather and his general health. After he completed his business, he suddenly noticed a sign by the check out desk that informed patients that they have an absolute choice as to what form of methadone they wish to receive, leaving him with the decided impression that he was a full and equal partner in his own care. Leaving the checkout desk, John suddenly remembered that he happened to have an appointment with his social worker that day. Appearing from around the corner to greet him, they walked together to his social worker's office.

After their appointment concluded, John's social worker requested a urine sample, something that is occasionally and randomly administered to all clinic clients. He accompanied him to the urine collection area, and handed John a cup with the relevant instructions on collection. John promptly provided the sample in a private, unmonitored bathroom and then gave it to his social worker who placed it in a bin for later processing.

John's social worker asked him if he'd like to see a psychiatrist that day in order to ensure that his medication regimen was working optimally for him, and John decided to take him up on the offer, as it was included in the cost of the treatment services provided, and available on site at this clinic. John made his way to his psychiatrist's office and made himself comfortable in the waiting room. After being invited in to the office, John had a brief interaction with the doctor, who renewed all of his prescriptions, including his prescription for a benzodiazepine to treat his anxiety disorder, before sending John on his way to enjoy the rest of his productive day. On the way out of the clinic, he noticed a familiar face in the waiting room and they exchanged jovial banter back and forth about whether the Cubs were finally going to make it to the World Series that year. This visit to the clinic was as untroubled and uneventful as every other visit John had ever experienced.

Later that year, John decided to pursue an advanced degree that entailed him moving out of state, and he began to make preparations. As an MMT patient, chief among his concerns were locating a new clinic in his new city, which happened to be Detroit. After locating the closest available clinic near his new environs, he found an apartment near the campus and got settled in.

On his first day in Detroit, he visited his new clinic for his intake. Upon arriving at the clinic, he noticed a group of what appeared to be clinic patients milling about the entrance, smoking cigarettes with dour looks on their faces. One of them gave John a friendly smile and a knowing nod as he entered the facility. The first impression that he received upon opening the door was the thick smell of must which permeated the air and the flicker of fluorescent lights that appeared to not have been changed for many years. The atmosphere was further depressed by the fact that layout of the waiting room looked like something that someone would find in a penal institution rather than in a medical facility.

The next bleak omen that only reinforced this impression was the fact that the front desk was not a front desk in as much as it is was a *hermetically sealed room* with foggy, *bullet-proof glass* separating the patients in the waiting area from the staff that manned the desk, from behind a locked *steel door*. Littering the glass partition were ominous threats and warnings posted by the staff for patients to read that dealt with all manner of clinic rules, regulations and dire warnings about what a patient could expect to happen should one fail to bring money to pay for their medication.

What further strengthened John's impressions of being in a penal institution was the double locked steel door that divided the clinic's offices from the waiting area. John noticed that the staff made quick entry and exit through this door via use of electronic key cards which they wore hanging from their necks. What John was really not prepared for beyond this dystopian presentation was the fact that the urine screening area of the clinic was located just behind this locked steel door and consisted of two bathrooms whose doors had built in windows so that the patient's "activities" could be fully monitored.

To further ensure monitoring ability, the bathroom's walls were almost entirely *mirrored*. The fact that the nursing staff that collected the urine samples was exclusively female did not seem to matter to anyone, but later in John's tenure at this clinic, it became clear that it mattered significantly to the male patient population. Humiliating was the first word that he often heard repeated, followed closely by dehumanizing. It felt to John that one was considered guilty of a crime one had never committed, and then punished by these demeaning procedures.

The clinic director finally appeared from behind the steel door and with a quick gesture that conveyed neither warmth nor welcome, he bade John to come back into his office. John followed the director down a series of dimly lit hallways in a building that had, in a different era, been known for its grandeur and opulence, but was reduced to a monument dedicated to perpetuating the misery of the humans it purported to serve. During their entire meeting, John was struck by the medical director's stoic affect, one *completely devoid* of friendliness or human affability. As John was to soon find out both from his personal interactions and the gossip among the patient population, it was more than just someone having a bad day, this was this gentleman's fundamental personality.

Unspoken, the doctor made it clear that he was un-amenable to even the most basic expressions of social grace, and this intake was the clinician's *best attempt* at a "meet and greet", to advise John of the clinic's policies and rules and to schedule John for his first meeting with a social worker. After this business was concluded, John was requested to provide a urine sample and had his first experience *urinating in front of a woman* who was not his intimate. The experience was psychologically unsettling, but John figured that since it was random, it wouldn't happen too often. He would be shortly disabused of that notion, as urine drops were *mandatory* from each patient *with each dosing*.

Stated differently, if you had to dose at this clinic every day (e.g. someone in their first several months of MMT), then *every day, before you were allowed to take your dose*, you first had to publicly urinate in front of an ever-so-watchful nurse. The amount of unnecessary stress imposed on the unfortunate patients is something that would be considered a "nonstarter" were we speaking of any other medical specialty. For the record, let it be noted that the federal regulations themselves require *eight* random urine screens *per calendar year*. (see Appendix I) As has been indicated before, no two MMT clinics in the U.S. operate in a singular, standardized, evidence-based manner. As such, they are "separate kingdoms unto themselves."

The juxtaposition between John's social workers, this one in Detroit and his former social worker in Chicago (who was *now* being remembered as a living saint,) was equally as stark, however not as brutal in presentation as the clinic director proved to be.

The most bizarre aspect of the clinic proved to be the dosing area, which consisted of one enormous bullet proof glass window that separated the patients from the single dispensing nurse, and instead of having a slot through which one could receive one's medication, there was a custom made lucite revolving door. This door was so striking because it was clearly *designed* so that there could be literally *no human contact* between nurse and patient. The nurses, not unlike the clinic director, extended no niceties or basic human kindness. Like an automaton, she dispensed the liquid methadone and observed as people would take it. With an expressionless face, she would shout through the bullet-proof rotunda, "O.K., you're done dosing? Leave."

The most distressing aspect of this entire experience was that the experiences at this clinic *never improved* in any way. There were so many hellish encounters that they all blurred into one another, making for one seemingly unending nightmare. Suffice it to say that an old adage was proved true: Humans treat other humans in the manner in which they expect them to behave, and sometimes, humans treat their fellow humans as if they did not possess the requisite humanity to be treated as such.

To understand the problems presented by this clear lack of quality control and standardization, we need to look at the effects that these deviations have on the clinic's patients, personnel and the communities which they serve. Arguably the single greatest danger to come from these variations lies in the realm of patient retention. A demoralized MMT patient is a patient that is one step closer to the (permanent) exit door, and as soon as MMT is discontinued, we know that the risk of relapse (and potential overdose) *skyrockets* and becomes that former patient's reality *again*. [131,132,133,138]

As it stands, there is so much confusion and controversy surrounding methadone maintenance that a sizable proportion of *patients themselves* are not fully clear on what is in their own best interest, meaning that because the clinics themselves often send the message, both implicitly and explicitly, that methadone is *not* a medication but rather it is simply to be considered and used as a *temporary* tool to ultimately wean oneself to abstinence, the number of relapses related to withdrawing from the clinic and overdose deaths is artificially high. This problem itself sometimes originates from the fact that many clinic personnel are themselves in a 12 step recovery program, so that their natural inclination is to guide people down the same path towards abstinence that they have taken.

The problem with this thinking, of course, is that what may have worked for one individual's addiction will likely not work for someone with a severe opioid addiction. This can lead to rapid demoralization in the patient, as the intrinsic message that they receive from counselors who rigidly adhere to the 12 step treatment mentality is that if they can't succeed at abstinence, *they* must somehow personally be at fault, or they must not have "wanted it" enough, when in reality nothing could be further from the truth.

This is the crux of the opioid addicted individuals current dilemma. They are caught between a rock, which is their addiction, and a very hard place which is the assortment and arbitrariness of the treatment modalities available to them at any given clinic. In all fairness, it is not the case that counselors actively force their clients towards an abstinence based solution, but rather that patients who are already suffering from low self esteem and a seriously bruised sense of self worth and efficacy can find themselves eagerly trying to please their counselors in order to gain some semblance of perceived approval and acceptance.

The solutions here are rather obvious. There must be a standardization of treatment protocols that codifies that methadone is to be used, unless otherwise indicated, as an end in itself. Only in exceptional cases should it be used as a means to some other end. The unfortunate reality is that we are still quite a ways off from being able to adopt these kinds of measures. Chief among the reasons for this lack of standardization originates with the

Federal Rules and Regulations regarding methadone. Implicitly, the regulations do appear to recognize methadone as a medication that is an end in and of itself, however, it's clear that this implicit message *must be explicitly codified* in order to allow for a much greater measure of standardization and acceptance.

What this would look like to an incoming patient would simply be that all of the risks and their actual options are explained up-front and in the clearest of terms. What are the risks? The clearest and most present danger is in the reality of relapse during any given period of abstinence and the potential for a lethal overdose during that relapse due to loss of tolerance. Furthermore, the statistics on relapse rates need to be made crystal clear, meaning offering 1, 3 and 5 year outcome data for MMT vs. abstinence based programs. Unfortunately, precisely these kinds of hard statistics are difficult to come by, mostly because there is little to no long-term (i.e. >1 year) follow-up of abstinence treated patients (of course, this shortage of information is, in no small part, due to the deep shame experienced by patients who relapsed from abstinence.) [138]

Were these numbers to be placed side by side in a bar chart form, the choice the patient would decide upon would be much easier to arrive at because one would see the abysmal relapse rates that abstinence-based treatment protocols produce for opioid addicted individuals. There will always be a small subset of patients who will *insist* that, *all evidence to the contrary*, they are going to go the abstinence route and that they will "make it." For this kind of personality, no amount of information will make a difference, but these people are relatively few and far between.

Most patients are simply looking to get better, to feel better, and to stop a crushing habit that has upended their lives and diminished their prospects. It remains axiomatic that at this point, at the beginning of the 21st century, properly executed MMT is the gold standard by which all other treatment modalities must be judged. [8,135]

As it stands today, MMT in the United States is really *only as good as the clinic from which one receives it*. Said another way, clinics that treat patients like infants and criminals cannot expect to have good outcomes for their patients. Conversely, when patients are treated with the same level of care and respect that patients who attend wound clinics or cardiovascular clinics or dialysis clinics are treated, good outcomes can be expected. People will often rise to the level of behavior which is expected of them, *ergo*, if you expect nothing but the worst, that is precisely the result you may expect to receive. It should go without saying, but it can't, that treating patients with kindness, compassion, and dignity should be an absolute prerequisite for care; however, since this is not the reality that patients enjoy at far too many MMT clinics, it has to be stated in black-and-white.

Methadone Maintenance Treatment is the only treatment modality that addresses the chronicity of opioid addiction. [8,135]

17

HOW TO TALK TO FAMILY AND FRIENDS

Carefully. Very Carefully. And with extreme prejudice. Though these statements may sound dramatic to some readers, they are actually merely representative of the status quo regarding MMT as it is *perceived* by the public. The experience of the vast majority of MMT patients who reveal their treatment status to friends and loved ones is so poor as to actually, *as a rule*, not be recommended. Of course, rules are made to have exceptions, and there will undoubtedly be cases wherein exceptions can be made; however, to reveal ones MMT status should in no way be undertaken lightly and without great forethought into the possible consequences of this disclosure. Remember, once the cat is out of the bag, it's out.

MMT still tends to be viewed by the public at large as being almost indistinguishable from heroin use itself since there is the commonly held myth that MMT is merely "substituting one addiction for another." This myth also leads to tremendous misinterpretations as to what methadone treatment really looks like and what it really entails. For example, many people, including members of law enforcement, seem to think that one can obtain a high from methadone and that this is the primary reason why it is taken. There appears to be no understanding of any of the treatment protocols, let alone the reasoning behind them.

This is an area which begs for continuing education training within the medical and law enforcement communities, as well as among public officials and legislators. As for what this further education would entail, most ideally, it would be presented at seminars from addiction specialists themselves who would disabuse individuals in positions of leadership of all of the myths, propaganda and stereotypes that presently exist and that inform their current discourse.

The very real and not to be minimized consequence of the disclosure of one's status is the potential for social ostracism. What this looks like is families and significant others refusing to speak with their children/relatives unless and until said children are *off* of methadone, because they are viewed as being "still on drugs." Friends will suspend further contact with the patient for fear of contamination and loss of status (mostly unconscious) and guilt by association.

The degree and brutality of this ostracism can best be likened to the social ostracism experienced by the very first HIV positive patients who eventually went on to develop full-blown AIDS, and how they were similarly *mistreated and abandoned* by friends and even their families of origin. This is simply history repeating itself. In reality the MMT patient, more than other people, *needs* contact with friends and loved ones so that this support system can help to buffer the stresses and strains that the MMT patient experiences by simply *having to live in the world as an opioid addicted individual/MMT patient.*

One must also be advised of the potential consequences of disclosure to an employer, as this can likewise produce a negative outcome. In terms of one's personal employment, the MMT elephant in the room generally should remain undisclosed unless there simply is no way to avoid it, which is the case when one is seeking employment that requires a drug screen. Different employers can have differing attitudes towards MMT, and there are many MMT patients who are successfully employed, so do not be misled into thinking that employment is a dead end pursuit if one is an MMT patient, as that is far from the case.

Should one unnecessarily disclose one's MMT status, anecdotally speaking, this *might* lead to an MMT patient suddenly being viewed as untrustworthy with merchandise or cash (irrespective of employment history,) and this is where potential negative ramifications, up to and including harassment and/or loss of employment, can develop. The great difficulty for MMT patients in this position is that they really have no realistic legal recourse, for while MMT patients do technically fall under the Americans with Disabilities Act (ADA), businesses are notoriously "flexible" in their adoption of the ADA's statutes, and since most MMT patients tend not to have the financial resources to hire an employment attorney, violations of the act can and do occur with impunity on a daily basis.

Before one chooses to disclose whether one is an MMT patient, or whether one is considering becoming one, ideally s/he should ascertain through indirect questioning what their loved ones think and know about MMT. Doing this allows him to tailor his approach more specifically to the situation at hand.

For example, if after questioning a loved one, they reveal that they believe that methadone is just substituting one addiction for another, one could then directly address this myth and dispel it with factual information. Ideally, it would help to be prepared with some pamphlets and books such as this that would further explain what MMT is so that the loved one is not left with the impression that the addicted individual is simply trying to justify their decision or "take the easy way out," whatever that is supposed to mean.

The importance of having actual physical references on hand cannot be overstated as these are essentially the liaison between your loved ones and MMT, bearing in mind that for most neurotypicals, *everything* that an addicted individual says is just a lie, as having an addiction often necessitates some dishonesty in order to keep the addiction going. Were addiction not _de jure_ illegal, there would be no need to lie.

It is important to note here that a loved ones response to your disclosure can have adverse consequences for you, up to and including said loved one's issuing ultimatums that involve everything from utilizing abstinence based treatment modalities (or else...) to literally ostracizing you from your family group or social circle.

This is why it is of the utmost importance that disclosure be made on an absolutely as needed basis, since the potential repercussions can be quite grievous. Bear in mind that information is power, and most importantly that *you* are equipped with the facts and all of the necessary information to make an informed decision; just be aware that your decision may not be supported by friends and family.

On a final note, this part is directed at friends, family, and significant others of a potential MMT patient, in other words, the ancillary neurotypical individuals around the opioid addicted individual.

Though you may not realize it, your support for a loved one entering MMT is vital to their recovery. While not being an absolute prerequisite for successful recovery in MMT, support from friends and family can go a long way toward making recovery in MMT resemble normal everyday life as possible, which is the most optimal atmosphere for an MMT patient.

For far too long, the opioid addicted individual has been ostracized and shunned by "normal" society, made to feel as if they were on the outside looking in. It would be a shame and a human tragedy if after being stabilized, the MMT patient were to still be shunned and ostracized, both because they need social connection to recover from their addiction as well as needing social connection in order to reclaim the human inter-dependence that has characterized our familial/tribal ancestors from the dawn of mankind.

Whether we like it or not, humans in general are far more inter-dependent than many modern people would care to acknowledge, and what that fundamentally translates into is the fact that we *need* each other in order to thrive. Yes, adult humans can and do survive under circumstances of isolation, sometimes even extreme isolation, but it is the rarest of individuals who *thrive* outside the company of others.

If your loved one is an MMT patient, or even just considering MMT as a treatment option, it is within your power to break the spell that is such a part of addiction, namely social ostracism and the attendant isolation of the addicted individual. It may be news to you, but addiction thrives where people are isolated and cut-off from their previous social bonds. This is why concepts like, "tough love" are entirely unhelpful (in the long-run) for opioid addicted individuals. They *already* are suffering tremendously, the last thing that is needed is for them to be proverbially kicked when they're already down.

Your man-on-the-street might be surprised by how much we, i.e. *homo sapiens sapiens*, *need* one another for our own health and happiness. This isn't about hippy-dippy ideas regarding love and peace; it is a tacit acknowledgment of the reality that humans *never* evolved as isolated beings, but rather, evolved in small groups (tribes, if you will) where survival alone was impossible and people *relied* on one another to simply gather the day's food supply.

That we are fundamentally social beings is actually encoded in our DNA, and it is our social selves that have advanced mankind beyond the level of small tribes. In case this talk of interdependence is making some readers uncomfortable, they would well be reminded that only centuries ago social ostracism was the equivalent of a death sentence, for the individual could not survive alone without the safety and security provided by the group.

The only difference is that today, people can quite literally survive without having any social connections whatsoever, but this is a kind of purgatory for the lone survivor because his internal need for social connectedness goes unanswered. In many ways, social disconnection is the new form of "banishment beyond the city walls."

If you are the loved one of a new MMT patient, please give that person a chance to actually thrive in MMT, instead of potentially floundering (and even dying) in abstinence, which is known to be ineffective in opioid addiction. Given enough time and the right tools, your MMT patient can be their old selves again, but they sure could use your support. Please give it to them. [138]

18

How to Make Methadone Maintenance Treatment Work for You

Should you choose to avail yourself of Methadone Maintenance Treatment (MMT), there are some general suggestions that can be made regarding how to make MMT work best for you personally. Recalling from previous chapters that addressed the inconsistencies between individual methadone clinics, [147] the first suggestion is to find a clinic and then, if one is geographically fortunate enough to live in a large urban area, to find a number of clinics and then do some homework as to what each individual clinic's mission statements are and what their particular treatment protocols look like.

The idea of choosing one's methadone clinic is presently still a luxury for most potential patients as many individuals do not live in large urban centers, let alone within close proximity to a methadone clinic. If one happens to be a person who lives a significant distance from any methadone clinic, wherein there is a dearth of methadone clinics, you will have fewer choices as to what kind of program you can attend. [147] That having been said, it is still important to emphasize that a poor methadone treatment facility is still better than no methadone treatment whatsoever.

The following advice is for all potential MMT patients at any given clinic.

Something that people may not initially consider is the importance of one's appearance and general affect, and arguably nowhere are these more important than when one is presenting themselves at a methadone clinic. By appearance, what is meant is quite literally one's external appearance, specifically in the form of hygiene, grooming and dress. One doesn't have to look like one just walked off the cover of a fashion magazine, but it really pays both in the short and long term to be meticulously groomed and well dressed.

Just to be clear, by well dressed, we are not referring to the latest fashion trends and fads, but rather the importance of simply wearing appropriate attire to the clinic. It is not uncommon for MMT patients to sometimes show up at a clinic in their bed clothes covered by perhaps nothing more a jacket. The message that this sends to anyone at the clinic is that this person is not being serious about their recovery, but more importantly, it undermines the clinic's trust in that individual as it concerns their treatment. This is particularly crucial in the later stages of MMT when one is potentially able to be granted take home privileges, *potential* being the operative word here. Another message that poor dress and grooming send to the clinic is that one's mental state is not stable and, once again, this cannot have any positive effect on one's current and future relationship with the methadone clinic.

Not too far behind in importance is one's affect. It, too, is an important factor in how one should present to the clinic. By affect, what is simply meant is the basic emotional appearance or the face that one shows the world. To not go to a clinic while intoxicated should be a given; what is more subtle are a suite of behaviors which are not uncommonly seen in a methadone clinic, particularly among patients early on in their treatment.

These behaviors can include, but are not limited to, confrontations with clinic personnel over perceived slights and unfair rules, open displays of emotion like frustration and anger, and sometimes simply context-inappropriate behaviors such as stepping out to smoke a cigarette when one is waiting for an appointment. The reason why the aforementioned can present problems is because it can very well happen that as the patient is outside smoking, their appointment is called and they are not present. Upon reentering the clinic and finding that one's appointment has been canceled or rescheduled simply because one was not immediately present could obviously lead to frustration and anger on the part of the patient, and this behavior could, in turn, be interpreted by staff as indicative of psychological instability or questionable reliability.

In short, behave and groom as if you are trying to impress. For an addicted individual who is in the early stages of their MMT, these suggestions may sound like a tall order or superfluous, however, experience has shown that these are indeed important factors that should not be ignored if one wants to have a positive MMT experience and a good relationship with ones MMT provider.

Though following these suggestions *may* seem difficult at first, bear in mind that what one is doing is not all that different from building a house. Every house requires a solid foundation in order to support the main structure and early on in MMT, first impressions and subsequent interactions serve as the laying of that foundation. If you are not taken seriously, you may not be treated seriously.

Closely related to the previous suggestions is the importance of punctuality and of showing up, period, when one is supposed to. Not feeling well enough to keep appointments is simply not an option for patients, as this only serves to undermine one's credibility and the assessment of ones character. If what is being said here comes across as paternalistic or patronizing, so be it, as in many ways, it is the current reality of MMT in the United States today, which dictates that a patient must do these things in order to obtain the most optimal treatment and treatment outcomes.

The reasoning behind this, while unfair, goes as follows: As an addicted individual entering a methadone clinic, one is already presenting as stigmatized, and it is unfortunately incumbent upon the patient themselves to dispel the myths behind the stigma.(see Chapter 19) The expectations that come with the stigma, in the form of each new patient who presents, are (by default) that the individual is unreliable, dishonest, untrustworthy, and unable or unwilling to control their basest impulses. Good grooming, punctuality and an appropriate affect can go a long way towards dispelling these stereotypes and can only serve to help the patient both in the short and long term.

As an MMT patient it is important to remember that one's reputation is not just important, it is everything in the eyes of the MMT provider. After all, once you have become an established, stabilized patient, their contact with you will be much less than in the early phase of treatment. Your reputation with your MMT provider is what helps them to decide what course of action to take with respect to your treatment plan, and it is foremost among things taken into consideration when treatment decisions are made. Guard and nurture your reputation as best you can.

One of the issues that you will encounter and find most trying during your early MMT experience is the need to exercise a great deal of patience, since by federal law, take home doses of methadone cannot even be considered until at least 90 consecutive days of drug free urine testing have been accumulated. Even after 90 days, it is important to remember that take home privileges are granted on a piece-meal basis, meaning that when one is first granted this privilege, one can only receive one to two take home doses per week and from there, with continued model behavior and negative urines, one can increase the number of doses that one is allowed to take home, which is only of benefit to the patient since fewer trips to the clinic are required, and one is thus freed to go back to work and to return to one's normal life.

The issue of take-homes is the single greatest potential problem for people attempting to enter MMT, and understandably so. The rules regarding take-homes are firmly ensconced in the federal regulations and they are very specific. In summary, each 90 days with no positive urines earns one a take-home bottle, up to the 180 day mark, at which point the provider *can* give the patient 6 take-homes per week. At the one year mark of consecutive "clean" urine tests, the provider *may* allow the patient up to a two week supply of take-homes, and at the two year mark of consecutive "clean" urines, the provider *may* allow for once-a-month take-home privileges. Depending upon the state one resides in, there may be some departures from this particular protocol in favor of less flexible, more strict take-home policies. This is one of the major problems with the federal regulations not being absolutely adhered to by individual states: A highly heterogeneous make-up of nation-wide MMT clinics. [147]

Obviously, this kind of dosing scheme can really wreak havoc for people who are steadily employed or seeking work just as they begin MMT. This is arguably the single greatest reason for people dropping-out of treatment early on: The clinic's federally mandated dosing schedule is almost prohibitive for many people with steady employment. There is no easy solution to this, unfortunately, so each person must do their homework as to how to make it feasible for them to *enter* MMT. The great irony, of course, is that once one has been in treatment for a while, this is no longer an impediment.

It is important to be aware that take home privileges are just that: privileges, and as they are given, they can also be rescinded, sometimes for reasons that can seem (and be) absolutely absurd. This is also why MMT clinics take the take-home regulations as a *suggested* time-line for granting take-homes. What *can* factor in very heavily into the take-home question are the patient's overall behavior, employment status, and most objectively, urine drug screen results. This is just yet another good reason to not use illicit drugs in MMT, and again, this is where discretion in choosing a clinic at the outset can help, if one is fortunate enough to be able to exercise that option.

In the best of all possible worlds, all MMT patients should eventually receive substantial take-home privileges, but in the real world there is always a not insubstantial fraction of patients at any given clinic without take-homes. Part of this has to do with the federal regulations for MMT patients in their first 6 months of treatment, part of it has to do with patients who have been there for longer than 6 months (sometimes substantially) but who continue to use street drugs on the side, and part of it has to do with the fact that take-homes are not *automatically* granted strictly according to the federal regulation's time-line.

If you find yourself unable to obtain take-homes because of continued illicit opioid use, by all means go to your provider and *request a methadone dose increase*, since it is highly likely that with enough methadone the extra drug intake will stop. And *always remember*, one person's "high dose" is another person's sub-therapeutic dose. This drives home the importance of individualized treatment and dosing plans.

At any given time your concern should not be focused on how high your dose is, but rather on *reaching a dose which will suppress any urges to use extra opioids.* Said another way, the focus should be on achieving *stability in treatment* and not on keeping your dose "low" so that your "eventual taper" will be quicker; this kind of thinking defeats the entire purpose of MMT and can result in early treatment failure.

It bears mentioning here that take home privileges are important and crucial for a sustained and strong recovery, but they also allow for the methadone maintenance patient to travel, even internationally. Should one require more doses than one is normally allotted for one's take homes, exceptions can be and are made for such travel, so reiterating, it really is in the best interest of the patient to have a good working relationship with their MMT clinic, counselors and doctors.

As to the very real subject of concurrent use of street drugs by the MMT patient, there are some serious words of warning here to avoid using any other street drugs (e.g. cocaine, pills, *ad infinitum*) for many reasons beside the obvious. The single most obvious reason to not concurrently use street drugs is because "positive" urines are often associated with a loss of take-home privileges. As can be clearly seen, most modern MMT employs both the carrot-and-the-stick to help patients stay on the "right path". Whether this is truly *ethical and appropriate*, not to mention therapeutic, still remains to be seen.

Since cocaine appears to be the most widely concurrently abused drug in MMT patients, it will be addressed directly in the following paragraphs, but bear in mind that what applies to cocaine applies to all other illicit drugs in a MMT context.

Illicit drug use during MMT can wreak havoc on one's progress in treatment by making it much more difficult for the provider to stabilize an MMT patient concurrently using cocaine, for a wide number of reasons. Perhaps at the top of the list of problems associated with cocaine use in MMT, cocaine can increase the rate at which the MMT patient metabolizes their daily dose, thereby putting them at risk for a relapse to illicit opioids. In addition, cocaine use puts the user at risk for potential arrhythmias, something that could prove disastrous considering methadone's known QT-interval prolongation. Cocaine, in general, is just a dead end drug.

Indirectly related to the above is the very real problem that is presented whenever one goes to the black-market for drugs: Drug dealers often sell more than just one kind of drug, and so temptation can be unnecessarily awakened in an otherwise stable MMT patient who is attempting to purchase 'only' cocaine. Add to this the fact that everything associated with the illicit procurement of drugs (i.e. people, places and things) is, in some way or another, toxic and detrimental to an MMT patient's recovery, placing the MMT patient at risk for adverse consequences from any of a number of sources – arrest by law enforcement and censure by one's MMT provider being the two most immediate ones.

A very serious warning about having run-ins with law enforcement while one is an MMT patient: In the U.S., almost no jails or prisons have any kind of ability (let alone willingness) to dispense *any* controlled medications whatsoever. This is still a very hairy situation, and with only a literal handful of correctional facilities that have recently been court-ordered to dispense methadone and psychiatric medications in the *entire country*, it is very strongly suggested that one stay on the absolute straight-and-narrow. [128]

To be clear, what is meant by this is that even something as civilian as accruing unpaid motor vehicle tickets *must be avoided at all costs*. Depending on your local jurisdiction, the police could put out a warrant for your arrest, and in a snap you could find yourself a resident of the county jail for 30 days because you were temporarily unable to pay the fine. *People have lost their lives this way*, often because they were on methadone and a benzodiazepine, or they were MMT patients with serious concurrent co-morbidities. [51,52,68,69,70,127]

Beware especially of jurisdictions where they can arrest you for unpaid parking tickets, and even if you don't live in such a jurisdiction, avoid parking tickets, period. Once one is caught up in the tentacles of the U.S. criminal justice system, it can be difficult (and sometimes impossible) to extricate one's self from it.

One more serious hazard must be addressed if we are to fully cover the dangers of combining MMT with any kind of incarceration. If you survive the cold-turkey withdrawal (if you're young and otherwise *healthy without*

any concurrent benzodiazepines or alcohol, you will in all likelihood survive jailhouse withdrawal) the prognosis for your survival *after release* is
not so great if you don't resume MMT. Whether you were on MMT before
you were incarcerated, or whether you just had a "street habit" at the time,
the time immediately after release is a highly risky period for former opioid addicted inmates. It is in the interest of your continued *survival* to go
(back) onto MMT. (129,130)

There is hope for the *future* for inmates who would require MMT.
Cases are slowly making their way through the courts, backed by a serious
and massive evidence-base, that would allow for U.S. correctional facilities to dispense controlled and psychiatric drugs. Since the wheels of U.S.
jurisprudence turn slowly, we would warn against excessive optimism on
this front, so until there is such a time for MMT in all jails and prisons
(and even thereafter) our advice is to just stay out of the arms of the law.
[128,130,131,132, 133,134]

Even the legal drug alcohol is something that is ideally best avoided,
when possible, by MMT patients, as excessive drinking is notorious for
speeding up the liver's metabolism of a dose of methadone, thus decreasing its effectiveness. Some MMT clinics will make selected patients use
a 'breathalyser' before allowing them to dose for that day, since some patients can be notorious drinkers. It happens on occasion that while waiting
in line to dose, one is sometimes literally hit by the overwhelming odor of
a distillery: This is because alcohol is excreted in the breath.

Some MMT patients clearly have a harder time stopping alcohol use
than do others, and if this describes you, a discussion with an addiction specialist (of which the clinic should have a number on hand) may be just what
the doctor ordered. If you have been drinking heavily for a while, ***do not***
attempt to stop on your own, as this may lead to dangerous, potentially lethal
withdrawal symptoms. Seek out an inpatient facility for safe withdrawal.

One issue that will not go away, at least for the foreseeable future, is
the question of *length of time* spent on MMT. In light of all the evidence
presented in this book, opioid addiction is the most tenacious addiction to
"beat" (i.e. remain abstinent from,) and this is something that currently is
not at all being emphasized by *any* media reports on the topic.

Perhaps, at least partially, it is for this reason that there are still MMT providers in the U.S. whose treatment philosophy is geared toward eventually tapering a patient's dose to zero so as to achieve *abstinence as the end-goal*. Still, considering all that has been learned over the past two decades regarding opioid addiction, one is at a loss to explain why this thinking persists among the very people who have been trained to treat addiction, MMT provider physicians.

Ultimately, each individual must make the *informed* decision of which path to take: Tapering to abstinence, or indefinite continuation of MMT. To contemplate indefinite continuation is to contemplate a life-time of MMT, and this is clearly something that demands heavy, serious thinking about this issue.

A few facts to bear in mind here; indefinite continuation MMT patients are indistinguishable from their neighbors precisely because the effective treatment of their opioid addiction has *finally* allowed them the opportunity to live the neurotypical life, for lack of a better phrase. Yet another example of how powerful language is, the author chooses to use the term indefinite continuation MMT in place of life-time MMT, as the latter term is too easily associated with potential negative memes such as, "life-sentence".

All of the years spent *not* being actively addicted to opioids, combined with reasonable take-home privileges (once-a-month,) has allowed these individuals to lay a solid foundation for their new life, and then build upon it, without the dangers of relapse, overdose, incarceration, etc. that tend to bedevil people who make attempts at abstinence. [138]

As even 12-step programs are forced to admit, abstinence (from opioids) is an extremely rare occurrence. Ultimately, attempted abstinence from opioids is, statistically speaking, akin to playing "Russian Roulette" with one's life. Without belaboring a point, the risk for relapse in an abstinent opioid addicted individual is so high that successful abstinence as the end-point is quite literally the exception, with recidivism being the rule.

The previous statement is *not* unprecedented, and in fact was made almost *100 years ago* by an experienced group of physicians.

"A *1926 report* to Britain's Ministry of Health examined the medical aspects of morphine and heroin addiction and *concluded that the prognosis for cure was poor*: "*Relapse, sooner or later, appears to be the rule and permanent cure the exception.*" [139] [ed. note: *emphasis added*]

The following quote best sums-up the different choices;
"Although methadone is sometimes used in a short-term detoxification protocol, *methadone has shown its best results when used as a long-term maintenance medication for opiate addiction.*" [140]

As a final note of caution, be wary of celebrities who had been addicted to opioids at some point in their lives but are now, ostensibly, "clean and sober" (Another good example of inappropriate language). One name that comes to mind, perhaps precisely because of his "star power," is Eric Clapton. He was once addicted to heroin, and now he is an abstinent, fervent 12-stepper. People can (and do) point to him as an example, saying, "Look, Eric Clapton did it, so you should also be able to." [78]

There are many confounding factors with respect to Eric Clapton's recovery, but what must be considered first and foremost is that Eric Clapton is an "uber-celebrity," with all of the attendant trappings of such social status. Money will *never* be a worry for E.C., neither will fear of not being able to afford medical services. Stated succinctly, E.C. does not face the very real *existential pressures* that all of the rest of us must confront on a daily basis. It's not hard to see how, within such a cocoon of a life, abstinence *may* actually be possible: Without all of the everyday stressors, relapse doesn't have much to feed upon. [78]

Just because person X is abstinent from opioids, and has been for many years, is not a reason to dismiss the very real risk of relapse that faces all opioid addicted individuals. We never know whether that person was ever *truly addicted* to opioids, or was an *excessive user* who wanted to stop. Your recovery is uniquely yours: Don't allow other people to overwhelm you with *their* dominant narrative. [78,138]

19

SOCIETAL STIGMATIZATION AND MARGINALIZATION OF THE ADDICT THE LANGUAGE OF MARGINALIZATION AND STIGMATIZATION

For most neurotypical readers, the concept that there could be an *active language of stigmatization* that marginalizes opioid addicts might seem counterintuitive, if not outright absurd. However, as will be demonstrated below, this is far from the case in real life.

The first thing that should be made clear is that the language of marginalization is not a direct one, which simply means that while nobody walks up to an opioid addicted individual and accuses him of being a scum sucking piece of shit, it is well-known that physicians used to frequently employ the acronym "S.P.O.S." when taking down patient notes regarding opioid addicts. S.P.O.S. stands for *Subhuman Piece Of Shit.* [18,19]

"No one deserves to be "treated like an addict," and it is outrageous that America's medical and legal systems have created a situation in which once addiction is suspected, compassion is eliminated. *There's no other disease where, after diagnosis, doctors simply drop patients for showing symptoms, all the while calling them despicable names*."

"And the irony is that treating addiction is far from the most difficult or hopeless task in medicine. While people in active addiction can admittedly sometimes be "hard to like," as Rutherford put it, people in recovery tend to be quite the opposite—and given time, **most people actually do recover**. [18] [ed. note: emphasis *theirs*]

While this is an extreme example of the language of marginalization, it is also substantially less common than the more typical everyday language that we hear in common usage – for example, how often does one hear the expression, "Johnny is finally 'clean'."? Clearly, the word "clean" implies that when Johnny *was* on drugs, he was no different than members of the "untouchable" caste in India – dirty, unholy, ungodly, and more frighteningly, *contagious*, as if the addicted individual was an infectious organism or vector for disease.

Equally disturbing is the use of the word "detoxification" in place of the more appropriate withdrawal. What is implied is that the person undergoing withdrawal is in a toxic state or even worse, they themselves are toxic and in need of "detoxification." There is definitely a pattern here, and that pattern involves the use of language that always, in some way, *besmirches* the opioid addicted individual's *character*. After all, wouldn't something "dirty" be in need of "detoxification"? Nowhere else in medicine is detoxification the word used to describe withdrawing people from medications *except* with respect to opioids.

Taken to its logical extreme, there is the belief that somehow just by association with lower-status individuals, one can lower their own status within society's hierarchical rungs. A tragic example of this is how often people will distance themselves from opioid addicted individuals who are open about their addiction status or treatment status in *any* way. This is such a common phenomenon that it can be considered to be essentially ubiquitous among addicts who choose to open themselves up to others without careful consideration of the potential consequences or risks involved.(see Chapter 17)

It is a sad reality that many an old friendship has been permanently destroyed by indiscriminate disclosure, and an even sadder reality that far too many families have been torn apart because of these memes that marginalize. [138]

Abstinence-based programs have a lot to do with this kind of stigmatizing language, whether intentionally or unintentionally, since their yardstick for successful recovery is a very narrowly defined one: Total and complete abstinence from *any and all* psychoactive substances *irrespective* of their true addictive potential.

For example, abstinence is very frequently advocated even for legitimate, psychiatrist-prescribed medications that do not fall under the mantle of addictive drugs, like antidepressants, certain anxiolytics, neuroleptic drugs, etc. The dangers that people face from prematurely discontinuing these kinds of medications at the behest of their 12-step brethren is rarely acknowledged, probably because to do so would be to admit that no matter the strength of ones 12-step brand of recovery, one is still no expert on medical (let alone psychiatric) issues. That this kind of discrimination is no different from the discrimination that the mentally ill so often face when they disclose their psychiatric status to friends, relatives and coworkers, is apparently lost on overly aggressive 12-steppers and others who *willfully choose* to maintain such negative attitudes towards MMT.

For all of these forms of stigmatization, the underlying dynamic *appears* to primarily have to do with the fear of being in the presence of someone who is believed to be not in full control of their own faculties, therefore somehow literally "infecting" or putting the neurotypical at risk of danger to their own personal or psychological integrity.

However, it will be news to many readers that there is a natural inborn protective mechanism in addicted individuals that prevents them from disclosing their addiction at precisely those times when they *might* be considered to be not in full control of their faculties: If the opioid addiction has not been "taken care of" ("fixed") or treated, the person will become so ill that they will avoid approaching a neurotypical person because they are terrified of literally being taken advantage of, as the addicted individual is at that time in a position of their greatest vulnerability and weakness.

These common, if diffuse, fears need to be recognized for what they are, namely the byproduct of decades of misinformation propagated as much by Hollywood films (such as The Basketball Diaries and Pulp Fiction) and the media as by the federal government itself in its relentless pursuit of opioid addicts, as if they were wanton criminals for whose problem the only solution is mass-incarceration and retribution. [20,23]

The federal government, in point of fact, has very intentionally pursued a campaign not only of misinformation but of disseminating disinformation regarding drugs. [20,23] Intentions are here entirely irrelevant, as the U.S. Federal Government's systematic campaign of disinformation has never produced anything even remotely positive from these "false flag" campaigns.

Generations of families have been destroyed by the false belief that Medication Assisted Treatment is not "real" recovery, and the criminal justice system is overloaded with people whose only "crime" is that they became severely addicted to opioids.

All of this because, "if a lie is told often enough it becomes truth," and isn't that were we have arrived? The addicted individual has become the villain and society's most convenient scapegoat for all manner of ills that have little (if anything) to do with drug addiction whatsoever, for example, decreasing academic performance nationwide, the deterioration of inner city neighborhoods most often brought about by "white flight," the ensuing collapse of the tax base and thus school funding, etc., etc.

The line from addiction to societal ills actually runs in the *opposite* direction. For example, a lack of living wage jobs makes for a dearth of two parent households, therefore, adult supervision of children is far less than what it used to be. Said children can, in turn, more easily become sidetracked or pipe-lined into activities that they would under normal circumstances never have participated in, such as drug use, robbery, petty theft, gang participation, etc.

Over and over again, we see this "reverse" line of causality (when compared to the dominant narrative) when it comes to drug addiction, with perhaps the clearest and most direct line of causality coming directly from the ACE's study. For example, the reader should be reminded that one need only accumulate four ACEs to be rendered 10x more likely to begin intravenous drug use. That's an increased risk of 1000% compared to controls, and so we see that early on in life the stage can be permanently set for a lifetime. [9,10]

To be more exact, the researchers discovered that for *each* ACE trauma that happens to a child, there is a corresponding two to four times greater likelihood that they will grow up to be an addicted adult. Remember, early trauma *consistently* produces, in a dose-dependent manner, increases in lifetime morbidity and mortality from all causes. This is a correlation so powerful that it is "of an order of magnitude rarely seen in epidemiology or public health." Translated simply, child abuse is as likely to cause drug addiction as obesity is to cause heart disease. There is tremendous predictive power in these studies. [23,27]

What can be seen most clearly from all of this is that the underlying pathology, if we must call it that, is something that is prodromally present *before* a person ever touches a drug. Healthy people tend not to abuse drugs whereas traumatized, vulnerable individuals have an increased risk of abuse and potential addiction, of this there can no longer be much doubt. (see Chapter 12)

The bottom line is that to blame and shame someone over their opioid addiction is the equivalent of blaming a schizophrenic for their disordered thinking: Nobody would dare blame the schizophrenic for something that is not their fault; the same should hold true for the opioid addicted individual.

For those last few hold-outs who insist that drug addiction, opioid addiction in particular, is the result of a personal choice, we would ask of these people one question: Going from the (false) assumption that addiction *is* a choice, we would ask these same people if they, "Felt it fair to be punished *for the rest of their lives* for singular indiscretions made at some earlier point in their lives?" Of course not.

Simply following that reasonable line of thought, why should the opioid addicted individual be "made to pay" for what was, potentially, *one* poor choice at some earlier point in their lives? Ironically, often enough the initiation into opioid use is *not* by choice but rather circumstance. If this thinking were *taken to its logical extreme*, we would spend inordinate amounts of time and money punishing anyone with a so-called "lifestyle" disorder: No more nicotine (ever...) for smokers, no more insulin for diabetics, no more healthcare for people who "just refuse" to lose the excess weight, no more anti-hypertensives for the non-compliant patient, and most certainly no more care for victims of lung cancer who were smokers.

That our everyday language is shot-through with examples of stigmatizing language is a painful reality: Whether referring to a positive urine drug screen as being a "dirty" drop, or insisting that someone on MMT is not truly "clean," this is a problem that is not likely to go away anytime soon. The best one can hope for is that with time, as information and education dispel the myths and stereotypes, most neurotypicals will begin to treat their MMT brethren as equals, and the good news is that this appears to be happening, albeit very gradually.

There will be one group to whom one can disclose without the fear of *social* repercussion, but ironically, this group would be health care professionals in general. This is not so much because healthcare professionals are any less susceptible to stigmatization and prejudice, but rather it is more a reflection of their desire to remain professional and detached at all times. The one warning here is that healthcare professionals can be *just as prejudiced* as your "man on the street," even though they should know better by dint of their professional training.

Generally speaking, disclosure to healthcare professionals *should* be done, if only to eliminate the potential for becoming labeled as a *"lying drug addict"* at some point in the future. With MMT, reputation is everything. As will be explained later, however, disclosure even to this group should be done cautiously.

An unfortunate reality is that even though the infamous S.P.O.S. designation among healthcare providers is still a fresh memory, and though it is now avoided for obvious reasons in written communications, one can never know what physicians and nurses *say* to one another. There is much reason to believe that not much has changed *except* for the fact that the dehumanization of opioid addicts no longer officially takes place in writing. As with racism, this form of prejudice has simply become more covert. [18,19,138]

A true Gordian Knot is presented by one situation that not infrequently confronts MMT patients: Whether or not to disclose one's MMT status to a treating psychiatrist. The reason why this is such a conundrum is because most psychiatrists are *terrified* of MMT patients abusing controlled substances, with the number one fear being prescription of a benzodiazepine to an MMT patient.

The bitter irony, of course, is that MMT patients suffer disproportionately from anxiety disorders and mood disorders, and thus are most often in a position to benefit from benzodiazepine co-prescription. The fear of accidental overdose and potential litigation appears to be so great with psychiatrists that they will often adopt a *one-size-fits-all rule of no benzodiazepines for MMT patients, irrespective of medical necessity.*

What this above scenario has resulted in is methadone providing physicians very often advising their MMT patients to *not* disclose their MMT status to psychiatrists, something that can "work" for the short-term, but is ultimately *disastrous advice* for MMT patients to follow in the long-run, for the following reasons; at some point, *sooner or later*, the MMT patient may have to check into a hospital for a medical emergency, and it is during these times that all of a patients' treating physicians are contacted so as to synchronize medical treatment. It is when physicians are being contacted that 'incidental information' such as MMT status can slip out.

When such an "informational" event happens with one's psychiatrist (to whom one had been lying, by omission, about MMT status,) it can and almost always does have a *devastating* effect on the doctor-patient relationship, as the psychiatrist will now become firmly convinced, via confirmation bias, that since his patient is really an MMT patient, his patient *must* be a pathological liar. In the matter of less than a minute, a good doctor-patient relationship where necessary benzodiazepines were provided can turn into an adversarial relationship where the MMT patient is now completely cut-off from their benzodiazepine prescription and effectively abandoned. Especially as of late, psychiatrists and other physicians have been "running for the hills," prescription pads firmly clutched in their hands.

This is one situation where each MMT patient will have to make a difficult choice that has no simple solutions as of now. A classic Catch-22 double-bind. For example, going to one's primary care physician *might* get one a benzodiazepine prescription, but for the reasons already mentioned, it most likely will *not* if you are a *known* MMT patient.

What is most frustrating about this particular reality is that one's actual standing as an MMT patient (i.e. as a long-term, stabilized patient in excellent standing) *appears to have no influence whatsoever on the outcome.* Whether you have been in MMT for 2 months or 20 years is entirely irrelevant (or, just too much effort) to too many U.S. physicians, methadone providers included and, likewise, your conduct as a patient (and human) can mean little-to-nothing in how you are treated by primary care physicians and other healthcare professionals. Once a move is made from one methadone clinic to another, for example, experience has shown that, unlike any other specialty, MMT providers are *entirely disinterested* in looking at your records from other clinics. [138]

The all-too-real result of this "horse-blinders" perspective on the MMT patient is that no matter if you have spent 8 years working hard on your good name and reputation, the minute you choose or have to go to another clinic, *it's as-if you were starting from square one* with respect to your reputation and patient history. This is another reason to choose your clinic (if you can) wisely, because you will want to stay at that one clinic for as long as is possible: Your good name and reputation are considered solely from *their* perspective, *not* from what another provider may have to say about you.

Add to this the contemporary reality that there is currently a benzodiazepine *hysteria* sweeping healthcare, and one can easily see how obtaining this potentially necessary medication can be extremely difficult for MMT patients. Few people actually lie with impunity, and fewer still want to be known for being dishonest, no matter the context. MMT patients are no different in this respect. [138]

This shows the persistent attitude both among professionals and the general public that addiction is a self inflicted vice, freely chosen in most cases, not a medically treatable disease. We are forced to ask, "Have we as a country become so jaded and cynical that we can in one fell swoop literally judge an entire heterogeneous group of people and, adding to this insult, then resolve that if they *must* be treated ethically, they must be put through the wringer?"

One study done in 2014 asked 1,010 primary care physicians in an anonymous web-based survey how they *personally felt* about people with Opioid Use Disorder (OUD) (a designation that they use for opioid addiction,) and the results were devastating;

"...displays respondents' beliefs about individuals with prescription OUD, and perceptions of the effectiveness of available treatments for opioid addiction. *Respondents reported high levels of desire for social distance:*

large majorities were unwilling to have a person with prescription OUD marry into the family (79%) or to work closely with the respondent on the job (77%). More than half (66%) viewed people with prescription OUD as more dangerous than the general population."

and

"We found that *larger proportions of physicians in our survey expressed negative attitudes toward people with prescription OUD than has the general public*, according to a nationally representative survey conducted on this topic in early 2014."

and

"74.4% [of respondents agreed with the statement,] '*Some people lack self-discipline to use prescription pain medications without becoming addicted*' [141,142]

Interestingly, this does raise the question of "if physicians are supposedly specialists in medicine, then why is it that when it comes to this medication, they literally 'need to go back to school' and either relearn, or learn something they've never been taught," either due to negligence on the part of medical school instructors or prejudice on the part of the medical student?

Ignorance of methadone and MMT may reach the level of a mentality where a doctor may simply think to himself, "I don't need to know this because I don't *plan* on having contact with this population group, and if they cross my path, I will rid myself of them as soon as possible and pass them off to the next physician." All of this, mind you, is completely legal. Said another way, in a more legalistic manner, these are the only forms of out-and-out patient neglect, patient abandonment, and medical malpractice that are *condoned* or are agreed upon *informally* as being acceptable protocol under the merciless scarlet letter of addiction. [138,141,142]

A troubling example of how maligned MMT is by the man-on-the-street's dominant narrative is to be seen (to be believed) in the alleged documentary movie released in 2005 with the title of "Methadonia." It is impossible to relay on paper the absolute reliance on confirmation bias that this movie has when it comes to depicting "a day in the life" of an "average" methadone patient, because it is *anything but*. This movie intentionally casts *only the treatment failures,* and then attempts to pass them off as, *"This* is methadone maintenance therapy," i.e., this is the norm for MMT, across the board.

It is hard to imagine a more *misleading and dishonest* depiction of MMT than the one presented by the movie "Methadonia." If the reader wishes to gain a picture of the massiveness of the stigma *against* MMT, we suggest that you watch this movie, but we also suggest that you be prepared: The entire film has been edited for maximum shock effect, and in this respect the movie resembles horror movies that rely heavily on a shock effect for the audience such as Dawn of the Dead, etc. The only thing missing from this movie besides integrity is honesty. The degree of stigmatization is literally *not to be believed.* [17]

Finally, we are going to be talking about the most destructive kind of stigmatization of all: Self-stigmatization. As has already been mentioned in this book, opioid addicts are no strangers to deeply internalized negative societal messages about their personal identity and image. A good number of the characters depicted in Methadonia display exactly this kind of self-loathing stigmatization.

Considering what is known about minorities internalizing the majority's negative stereotypes and beliefs, it should come as little surprise that opioid addicted individuals often struggle with their sense of self. This manifests itself most detrimentally in MMT patients who have internalized the negative dominant narrative regarding methadone as a medicine; it's no wonder that a substantial number of MMT patients are "repeat customers," if they survive relapse, simply because they are *obsessed* with the idea of using methadone to taper down to abstinence, never accepting that they might very well be unable to *sustain* abstinence.

A study of 393 primary care patients diagnosed with Opioid and Alcohol Use Disorders (OAUDs) (but not in treatment) were given several questionnaires relating to different aspects of their OAUDs. What follows is a synopsis.

"The majority of participants reported thinking, at least sometimes, that they "have permanently screwed up" their lives (60%), and felt "ashamed" (60%), and "out of place in the world" (51%) as a result of their opioid or alcohol use. Higher internalized stigma was significantly related to more substance use problems."

"...our results suggest that internalized stigma might be related to negative outcomes for primary care patient population coping (*sic*) with OAUDs [Opioid and Alcohol Use Disorders.] It is plausible that strong self-identification with negative stereotypes, among some individuals representing this stigmatized population, might hinder their ability to cope with negative consequences of substance use."

Perhaps most troubling of all was the finding that 44% of respondents endorsed the following statement, "I feel inferior to people who have never had a problem with substances," while a full 47% endorsed this statement, "I have the thought that I can't be trusted." [143]

These are tragic numbers reflecting the self-stigmatization of people with opioid addiction and/or alcoholism. They are clearly high enough that they provide a lot of explanatory power to why so many opioid addicted individuals, even those in MMT, succumb to the *lethal siren song* that their own society is singing, a song whose origins can be traced all the way back to the beginnings of the Prohibition on opioids at the turn of the last century. It is a siren song in that it sends the unequivocal message that *only* total abstinence is an acceptable outcome for the opioid addicted individual. [17,135,138]

It's been long overdue that the message of utter contempt for opioid addicts that Harry Anslinger single-handedly crafted must die, along with the antiquated and blatantly unsuccessful ideas that he endorsed with respect to opioid addiction. No enlightened physician of today would knowingly agree with Anslinger's motives and methods, so why are they still so overrepresented among the lay population and other healthcare professionals? [23,61]

It is argued here that there has been an appalling lack of frank, honest information about drugs in general and opioids specifically. As of this writing, there are public service announcements (PSA's) claiming that, "opioid drugs can cause *dependence* in 5 days," which, strictly speaking, is correct. [144] What is *left out* of the commercials is the fact that *addiction* usually takes substantially longer to set in, *and* one must have an underlying set of vulnerabilities for this process to occur.(see Chapters 11, 12)

Seriously, what makes people in any position of authority think that they are going to prevent addiction by *lying* to people, or "distorting" the facts? It hasn't worked for the past century: Why would it, all-of-a-sudden, work now?

20

SIDE EFFECTS OF METHADONE,
AND WHAT TO DO ABOUT THEM

While methadone is generally well-tolerated by most people, there are some side-effects which can, depending upon one's individual physiology, be distressing. Most side-effects abate or get better with time, while some may require some more long-term responses.

Initially, during the induction phase and during the first months, some sedation may be present particularly in the hours immediately after dosing for the day. This sedation disappears with time at a steady, stabilizing dose.

Without a doubt the most common complaint about methadone side effects has to do with the constipation produced by this medication, as all opioids have a constipating effect. Because of methadone's long duration of action, this constipation *can* be quite severe, particularly during induction and the first months of MMT. As such, it is nearly universally recommended by treatment providers that the early MMT patient incorporate a regimen of stool softeners, increased fiber in the diet, and increase one's water intake. Together, these measures themselves usually suffice to keep things moving, but if they don't, there are still many options available for the MMT patient with recalcitrant constipation.

Before proceeding any further, let's make sure that any potential confusion regarding this issue can be minimized, and in keeping with the structure of this book, we will do so by presenting clear and concise, evidence-based information. The disclaimer here is that, for some people at least, discussions about bowel habits can be "off-putting," and therefore this is one context where our more sensitive readers may need to push through the rest of this chapter with gritted teeth; this information is unavoidably *necessary*.

One very common misunderstanding concerns the difference between stool softeners and laxatives. To many laypersons these two things are understood as being one and the same thing, just expressed differently. In reality, they are two different classes of medication that are used to accomplish different therapeutic ends. Of great importance to the MMT patient, these differences *do* matter, and it is critical that the new MMT patient understand them.

Stool softeners, the main medications we are referring to here, are agents that do exactly as their name implies, namely make a given mass of stool softer and more malleable. That is all that they do. Unlike laxatives, they do not increase the frequency of bowel movements, as they do not exert a laxative effect, they only change the consistency of the stool.

Unless you require them, we recommend that you stay away from anything resembling regular use of laxatives. They will only cause trouble when used excessively, and can even produce dangerous electrolyte imbalances if abused. That being said, they may be required on rare occasions for rather exceptional reasons.

Stool softeners, on the other hand, are often a mainstay of an MMT patient's medication regimen. Whether one will require stool softeners indefinitely (they are not habit-forming, unlike laxatives) will really depend upon a given MMT patient's personal physiology. Some people are more sensitive to the constipating effect of opioids than are others. When in doubt, a quick discussion with your MMT physician should clarify any questions.

Of the available OTC stool softeners, docusate sodium (a.k.a. Colace) is the one most often used by MMT patients. They come in 100 mg softgel capsules and should ideally be taken with meals. As to the precise dose per meal, this will have to be determined by each individual, but one capsule per meal is a good dose to start with. Docusate sodium can be very cheaply purchased from warehouse clubs like Costco. The next cheapest place would be "dollar" stores.

Occasionally, one might come across docusate *calcium* (a.k.a. Surfak,) but this is just a much more expensive version of docusate sodium, and does not differ otherwise. Unless it happens to be cheaper than Colace, there is no advantage conferred by its preferential use. Docusate works by acting as a surfactant for the stool, similar to how dishwashing liquid increases the "wetting" power of dirty wash water.

There may be times, depending on the MMT patient's personal medication regimen and lifestyle, when mere stool softening is not enough. It is during these times that the use of a mild laxative such as bisacodyl (Dulcolax) can help, just be sure to strictly follow the package instructions.

There may also be times when a stool-softener is not enough, but a laxative is too much. It is for these intermediate periods of constipation that we recommend polyethylene glycol 3350 (a.k.a. Miralax,) since it provides a happy medium between the two. The way it works is that it is a powder that dissolves in water but does not penetrate the intestinal lining, causing a net-effect of pulling water from outside into the intestine where it can moisturize an otherwise dry stool. Miralax can have a slight laxative effect, due to it's osmotic effects in the human intestine, but it is not a habit-forming laxative in the strict sense and so can be safely used over longer periods, if necessary. The usual dose is one "cap full" of powder to 4-6 oz. of liquid, to be stirred and then taken with or without meals.

Like generic Colace, generic Miralax can also be most cheaply purchased from warehouse stores like Costco and then next cheapest would be Target.

A substantially less irksome side-effect of methadone that also occurs most often during induction and early treatment is a slight feeling of tiredness at some point in one's dosing "cycle," but this side effect usually resolves by itself with enough time in treatment.

Excessive sweating sometimes occurs in MMT patients, and this is an effect that may or may not resolve with time.

Because of potential effects on the hypothalamic-pituitary-gonadal axis, some MMT patients *may* experience changes in libido, usually a reduction. Treatment of this particular side-effect, when present, may or may not require some testosterone replacement therapy in men, particularly in men > 40 years of age. This particular side-effect appears to be highly individualized, with some patients reporting reduced libido and others reporting no such effect. If you experience *bothersome* changes in libido, a discussion with a primary care physician and your MMT provider may be a good idea.

One potential side effect of methadone that will not be detected by the MMT patient themselves is a cardiac phenomenon known as QT-interval prolongation. This effect, which is also a side effect of a vast number of other prescription medications is, *generally speaking*, harmless. That having been said, this is one of the reasons why it is so important to be completely open about one's general medical history with MMT providers. There are a very small minority of patients, usually with congenital heart issues, for whom methadone would be contraindicated as it could provoke a potentially deadly cardiac arrhythmia known as torsades de pointes. [145]

Nowadays, it would be exceptional to find a methadone provider in the U.S. that does *not* order an electrocardiogram (EKG) as part of the initial intake physical work-up. Since this has become common practice, it is now essentially impossible to fall through the cracks, so to speak, because risk for torsades de pointes due to methadone can now be immediately assessed. So to sum it up, QT-interval prolongation is a side effect of methadone, but as with so many other medicines that share this property, it is of little practical consequence to the would-be MMT patient.

Because methadone can prolong the QT-interval, it is important for the MMT patient to talk to their provider if they are being prescribed a new medication from a different physician, as one wants to avoid using *multiple* QT-prolonging medications *together* for the above stated reasons. When in doubt, ask your healthcare or MMT provider which (if any) of your medicines can cause QT-interval prolongation. [145]

One final word about side effects: There is one side-effect that does not diminish nor disappear with time, and that effect would be what is known as pupillary miosis, or in plain english, constricted pupils. If you are a person with dark irises, then this is not much of a potential issue, as the constricted pupils can only be seen against a light background.

If you are a person with light-colored eyes (e.g. blue, green, hazel, etc.) this side-effect may, and the emphasis here is on *may*, be noticed by a neurotypical as they are speaking with you. The lighter the color of the iris, the more noticeable it is.

The degree of constriction can be quite extreme, which is why it is being mentioned here: As an MMT patient, it probably makes sense to have a stand-by "excuse" for one's constricted pupils if one has light colored eyes, since some (very, *very few*) people *may* ask in an entirely harmless manner why your eyes look like they do. What you tell them is entirely up to you, just make sure that what you say is at least somehow rooted in truth, since part of MMT consists of the patient being honest to themselves as well as others (wherever possible.)

This particular point about being prepared for questions about "why are your pupils so tiny?" is not so much made because the question is frequently asked (it's not,) but instead to point out both the importance of the MMT patient having a full awareness of what is going on in their body as well as emphasizing that in MMT, it makes realistic sense to be prepared for the occasional odd question.

One particular property of methadone that is not a side-effect, but that requires stating, is that methadone is not harmful or injurious to any human organs or body systems, even when taken over a period of decades. Unlike alcohol, methadone does no permanent damage to the body. [29] Something which must be stated for the record is that opioids, as a class of medications, are non-toxic to the human body even after protracted periods of use.

The diseases and disability incurred by the illicit use of opioids have nothing to do with any pathogenic quality that they possess, since they are non-pathogenic. All of the diseases and physical infirmities created by illicit opioid use have their origin in the very fact that they are illegal, with all of the attendant sequelae being a direct result of people obtaining their opioids from the unregulated black-market. It should go without saying that criminals do not care about things like quality control, precise dosages, or purity, etc.

Any objective, informed observer would come to the above conclusion, since it is reflective of the *realities* confronting opioid addicted individuals. In the most honest and objective analysis, it is not opioids themselves that are vectors for disease, but rather their illegality creating a perfect storm of confluence of circumstance to create such terrible (and sometimes, irrevocable) damage and inflict so much suffering unnecessarily. [18,138]

21

MEDICATIONS TO AVOID WHEN ON MMT

This can be a problematic issue for some patients maintained on MMT, as many patients have concurrent psychiatric and/or medical issues that also require medications. First and foremost, avoid any and all opioid antagonists, be they full or partial antagonists. A good example of full antagonists would be naltrexone, nalmefene and, unless you're in danger of an overdose, naloxone.

Of these three, naloxone and nalmefene are the easiest to avoid because naloxone doesn't work orally, and nalmefene is available as an injection only. Naltrexone can be a danger, because it is also marketed as an anti-drinking pill for alcoholics under the trade name Revia, among others and generics. Be forewarned, one naltrexone tablet can land an MMT patient in the E.R, with withdrawal so severe that the affected individual has to be placed in the I.C.U.

The partial antagonists are more tricky, since one of them is actually marketed as an alternative to methadone, namely, buprenorphine. Too many anecdotes abound of stabilized MMT patients, curious about Suboxone, winding-up in the E.R. in induced (a.k.a. precipitated) withdrawal. The bottom line is, if you are an MMT patient, avoid Suboxone (or its equivalents) at all costs. As with naltrexone, once the withdrawal sets in (rapidly,) it can be very difficult to override/reverse for >24 hours.

Of the other partial antagonists, the one still relatively widely in circulation as a mild pain reliever is pentazocine, a.k.a. Talwin. The others worth mentioning, just to cover all of our bases, are butorphanol and nalbuphine. If you are an MMT patient or you have a need for illicit opioids, stay away from these medicines. They can all precipitate a severe withdrawal syndrome in MMT patients.

Barbiturates in general are extremely contraindicated because barbiturates are all promiscuous inducers of the liver cytochrome P450 enzyme system. As such, when we speak of enzyme induction, what we are referring to is the opposite of enzyme inhibition. Enzyme inducers *increase* the rate of the synthesis and turnover of the CYP450 enzyme in the liver. A person taking a barbiturate concurrently with methadone will, depending on the barbiturate, sooner or later, precipitously go into withdrawal because the induced-enzyme will "burn through" the methadone, vastly increasing the rate of its metabolism.

What may have been a perfectly effective holding dose can all of a sudden leave the patient in a state of severe withdrawal only hours after taking it. Of the barbiturates, the number one to be avoided is phenobarbital because it is *such* a potent inducer across the board of all liver enzymes that in fact it is used in laboratory research to effect that very change. Phenobarbital is still used to this day rather widely as an antiseizure medication.

Phenytoin (Dilantin) and primidone, both anti-seizure drugs, also have almost as potent a level of liver enzyme induction as does phenobarbital.

Carbamazepine, another anti-seizure medication, is another drug to be avoided for the same reason. There are many other anti-seizure medications that do not induce CYP450 enzymes, one example being divalproex sodium (Depakote).

Rifampin, an anti tuberculosis drug, and a large number of the HIV anti-retro-viral drugs also have the capacity to induce liver enzymes. This level of induction may or may not be as aggressive as the aforementioned drugs, but if necessary, a methadone dose-increase may very well be needed to prevent breakthrough withdrawal signs.

In general, the important thing to remember is to think anti-epileptic, anti-retroviral, anti-tuberculosis, and possibly certain chemotherapeutic agents. This is where the doctor-patient relationship is so crucial but, unfortunately, precisely because of the destructive stigmatization of and prejudice against addicts across the board, this relationship is far too often compromised by stigma on the part of the physician and internalized stigma on the part of the patient. It is not uncommon to hear physicians make absurd remarks like "x number of milligrams should be more than enough methadone for anyone."

Often times what is a sufficient dose in a stabilized MMT patient will become an insufficient dose if taken with certain liver enzyme-inducing drugs, and this is what is crucial to bear in mind: If you have to take an enzyme inducer, then make sure to get a corresponding increase in your methadone dose according to your symptoms. A short discussion with the methadone provider *should* be all that it takes to get that ball rolling.

Another potential issue with methadone treatment is known as QT-prolongation, and it is something that occurs to some degree in all patients receiving methadone, some more so than others. For the most part, this is a silent, harmless side-effect for most patients, however, here again we see the luck of the genetic draw playing a big role: A very small number of people have what is known as prolonged QT-syndrome, and in these patients methadone may produce a potentially fatal cardiac arrhythmia known as torsades de pointes. For this reason, EKG (electrocardiogram) testing is now almost routine for all potential (and even some current) MMT patients.

EKG testing can screen out those patients at risk of QT-prolongation, but QT-prolongation may also occur in stabilized MMT patients who are prescribed certain, more esoteric drugs than the ones listed above. A full list of these QT-prolonging medications is outside the scope of this book as it would take up an inordinate amount of space (there are so many,) but a conversation with one's doctor or a pharmacist will help to clear up any potential questions regarding what medications to avoid. [145]

The great equalizer in all of this lies in the fact that all of the information that is now available to the general public is vastly more informative and helpful than that which was available at the turn of the last century. A century of absolute and utter social ostracism, blaming, and dehumanization has made most opioid addicted individuals extremely guarded in their interactions with medical personnel. [138]

If you don't feel comfortable talking to a physician or a pharmacist about this issue, there are entire lists of QT-prolonging drugs on the internet for anyone to peruse. Just be careful to get your information from a reliable source and when in doubt, double-and-then-triple-check it.

The truest meaning of liberty...where individuals simply have, as their birthright, the ultimate right to make choices for themselves, they're certainly always held accountable, so they should have the right to pursue whatever means are necessary for them to be happy. Keeping this in mind, we have to remember that happiness is in the eye of the beholder...

APPENDIX I

Title 42 Code of Federal Regulations
Section 8.12 – Federal opioid treatment standards.

§ 8.12 Federal opioid treatment standards.

(a) *General.* OTPs must provide treatment in accordance with the standards in this section and must comply with these standards as a condition of certification.

(b) *Administrative and organizational structure.* An OTP's organizational structure and facilities shall be adequate to ensure quality patient care and to meet the requirements of all pertinent Federal, State, and local laws and regulations. At a minimum, each OTP shall formally designate a program sponsor and medical director. The program sponsor shall agree on behalf of the OTP to adhere to all requirements set forth in this part and any regulations regarding the use of opioid agonist treatment medications in the treatment of opioid use disorder which may be promulgated in the future. The medical director shall assume responsibility for administering all medical services performed by the OTP. In addition, the medical director shall be responsible for ensuring that the OTP is in compliance with all applicable Federal, State, and local laws and regulations.

(c) *Continuous quality improvement.*
(1) An OTP must maintain current quality assurance and quality control plans that include, among other things, annual reviews of program policies and procedures and ongoing assessment of patient outcomes.

(2) An OTP must maintain a current "Diversion Control Plan" or "DCP" as part of its quality assurance program that contains specific measures to reduce the possibility of diversion of controlled substances from legitimate treatment use and that assigns specific responsibility to the medical and administrative staff of the OTP for carrying out the diversion control measures and functions described in the DCP.

(d) *Staff credentials.* Each person engaged in the treatment of opioid use disorder must have sufficient education, training, and experience, or any combination thereof, to enable that person to perform the assigned functions. All physicians, nurses, and other licensed professional care providers, including addiction counselors, must comply with the credentialing requirements of their respective professions.

(e) *Patient admission criteria* -
(1) *Maintenance treatment.* An OTP shall maintain current procedures designed to ensure that patients are admitted to maintenance treatment by qualified personnel who have determined, using accepted medical criteria such as those listed in the Diagnostic and Statistical Manual for Mental Disorders (DSM-IV), that the person is currently addicted to an opioid drug, and that the person became addicted at least 1 year before admission for treatment. In addition, a program physician shall ensure that each patient voluntarily chooses maintenance treatment and that all relevant facts concerning the use of the opioid drug are clearly and adequately explained to the patient, and that each patient provides informed written consent to treatment.

(2) *Maintenance treatment for persons under age 18.* A person under 18 years of age is required to have had two documented unsuccessful attempts at short-term detoxification or drug-free treatment within a 12-month period to be eligible for maintenance treatment. No person under 18 years of age may be admitted to maintenance treatment unless a parent, legal guardian, or responsible adult designated by the relevant State authority consents in writing to such treatment.

(3) *Maintenance treatment admission exceptions.* If clinically appropriate, the program physician may waive the requirement of a 1-year history of addiction under paragraph (e)(1) of this section, for patients released from penal institutions (within 6 months after release), for pregnant patients (program physician must certify pregnancy), and for previously treated patients (up to 2 years after discharge).

(4) *Detoxification treatment.* An OTP shall maintain current procedures that are designed to ensure that patients are admitted to short- or long-term detoxification treatment by qualified personnel, such as a program physician, who determines that such treatment is appropriate for the specific patient by applying established diagnostic criteria. Patients with two or more unsuccessful detoxification episodes within a 12-month period must be assessed by the OTP physician for other forms of treatment. A program shall not admit a patient for more than two detoxification treatment episodes in one year.

(f) *Required services* -
(1) *General.* OTPs shall provide adequate medical, counseling, vocational, educational, and other assessment and treatment services. These services must be available at the primary facility, except where the program sponsor has entered into a formal, documented agreement with a private or public agency, organization, practitioner, or institution to provide these services to patients enrolled in the OTP. The program sponsor, in any event, must be able to document that these services are fully and reasonably available to patients.

(2) *Initial medical examination services.* OTPs shall require each patient to undergo a complete, fully documented physical evaluation by a program physician or a primary care physician, or an authorized healthcare professional under the supervision of a program physician, before admission to the OTP. The full medical examination, including the results of serology and other tests, must be completed within 14 days following admission.

(3) *Special services for pregnant patients.* OTPs must maintain current policies and procedures that reflect the special needs of patients who are pregnant. Prenatal care and other gender specific services or pregnant patients must be provided either by the OTP or by referral to appropriate healthcare providers.

(4) *Initial and periodic assessment services.* Each patient accepted for treatment at an OTP shall be assessed initially and periodically by qualified personnel to determine the most appropriate combination of services and treatment. The initial assessment must include preparation of a treatment plan that includes the patient's short-term goals and the tasks the patient must perform to complete the short-term goals; the patient's requirements for education, vocational rehabilitation, and employment; and the medical, psychosocial, economic, legal, or other supportive services that a patient needs. The treatment plan also must identify the frequency with which these services are to be provided. The plan must be reviewed and updated to reflect that patient's personal history, his or her current needs for medical, social, and psychological services, and his or her current needs for education, vocational rehabilitation, and employment services.

(5) *Counseling services.*
(i) OTPs must provide adequate substance abuse counseling to each patient as clinically necessary. This counseling shall be provided by a program counselor, qualified by education, training, or experience to assess the psychological and sociological background of patients, to contribute to the appropriate treatment plan for the patient and to monitor patient progress.

(ii) OTPs must provide counseling on preventing exposure to, and the transmission of, human immunodeficiency virus (HIV) disease for each patient admitted or readmitted to maintenance or detoxification treatment.

(iii) OTPs must provide directly, or through referral to adequate and reasonably accessible community resources, vocational rehabilitation, education, and employment services for patients who either request such services or who have been determined by the program staff to be in need of such services.

(6) *Drug abuse testing services.* OTPs must provide adequate testing or analysis for drugs of abuse, including at least eight random drug abuse tests per year, per patient in maintenance treatment, in accordance with generally accepted clinical practice. For patients in short-term detoxification treatment, the OTP shall perform at least one initial drug abuse test. For patients receiving long-term detoxification treatment, the program shall perform initial and monthly random tests on each patient.

(g) *Recordkeeping and patient confidentiality.*

(1) OTPs shall establish and maintain a record keeping system that is adequate to document and monitor patient care. This system is required to comply with all Federal and State reporting requirements relevant to opioid drugs approved for use in treatment of opioid use disorder. All records are required to be kept confidential in accordance with all applicable Federal and State requirements.

(2) OTPs shall include, as an essential part of the record keeping system, documentation in each patient's record that the OTP made a good faith effort to review whether or not the patient is enrolled any other OTP. A patient enrolled in an OTP shall not be permitted to obtain treatment in any other OTP except in exceptional circumstances. If the medical director or program physician of the OTP in which the patient is enrolled determines that such exceptional circumstances exist, the patient may be granted permission to seek treatment at another OTP, provided the justification for finding exceptional circumstances is noted in the patient's record both at the OTP in which the patient is enrolled and at the OTP that will provide the treatment.

(h) *Medication administration, dispensing, and use.*

(1) OTPs must ensure that opioid agonist treatment medications are administered or dispensed only by a practitioner licensed under the appropriate State law and registered under the appropriate State and Federal laws to administer or dispense opioid drugs, or by an agent of such a practitioner, supervised by and under the order of the licensed practitioner. This agent is required to be a pharmacist, registered nurse, or licensed practical nurse, or any other healthcare professional authorized by Federal and State law to administer or dispense opioid drugs.

(2) OTPs shall use only those opioid agonist treatment medications that are approved by the Food and Drug Administration under section 505 of the Federal Food, Drug, and Cosmetic Act (21 U.S.C. 355) for use in the treatment of opioid use disorder. In addition, OTPs who are fully compliant with the protocol of an investigational use of a drug and other conditions set forth in the application may administer a drug that has been authorized by the Food and Drug Administration under an investigational new drug application under section 505(i) of the Federal Food, Drug, and Cosmetic Act for investigational use in the treatment of opioid use disorder. Currently the following opioid agonist treatment medications will be considered to be approved by the Food and Drug Administration for use in the treatment of opioid use disorder:

(i) Methadone;

(ii) Levomethadyl acetate (LAAM); and

(iii) Buprenorphine and buprenorphine combination products that have been approved for use in the treatment of opioid use disorder.

(3) OTPs shall maintain current procedures that are adequate to ensure that the following dosage form and initial dosing requirements are met:

(i) Methadone shall be administered or dispensed only in oral form and shall be formulated in such a way as to reduce its potential for parenteral abuse.

(ii) For each new patient enrolled in a program, the initial dose of methadone shall not exceed 30 milligrams and the total dose for the first day shall not exceed 40 milligrams, unless the program physician documents in the patient's record that 40 milligrams did not suppress opioid abstinence symptoms.

(4) OTPs shall maintain current procedures adequate to ensure that each opioid agonist treatment medication used by the program is administered and dispensed in accordance with its approved product labeling. Dosing and administration decisions shall be made by a program physician familiar with the most up-to-date product labeling. These procedures must ensure that any significant deviations from the approved labeling, including deviations with regard to dose, frequency, or the conditions of use described in the approved labeling, are specifically documented in the patient's record.

(i) *Unsupervised or "take-home" use.* To limit the potential for diversion of opioid agonist treatment medications to the illicit market,opioid agonist treatment medications dispensed to patients for unsupervised use shall be subject to the following requirements.

(1) Any patient in comprehensive maintenance treatment may receive a single take-home dose for a day that the clinic is closed for business, including Sundays and State and Federal holidays.

(2) Treatment program decisions on dispensing opioid treatment medications to patients for unsupervised use beyond that set forth in paragraph (i)(1) of this section, shall be determined by the medical director. In determining which patients may be permitted unsupervised use, the medical director shall consider the following take-home criteria in determining whether a patient is responsible in handling opioid drugs for unsupervised use.

(i) Absence of recent abuse of drugs (opioid or nonnarcotic), including alcohol;

(ii) Regularity of clinic attendance;

(iii) Absence of serious behavioral problems at the clinic;

(iv) Absence of known recent criminal activity, e.g., drug dealing;

(v) Stability of the patient's home environment and social relationships;

(vi) Length of time in comprehensive maintenance treatment;

(vii) Assurance that take-home medication can be safely stored within the patient's home; and

(viii) Whether the rehabilitative benefit the patient derived from decreasing the frequency of clinic attendance outweighs the potential risks of diversion.

(3) Such determinations and the basis for such determinations consistent with the criteria outlined in paragraph (i)(2) of this section shall be documented in the patient's medical record. If it is determined that a patient is responsible in handling opioid drugs, the dispensing restrictions set forth in paragraphs (i)(3)(i) through (vi) of this section apply. The dispensing restrictions set forth in paragraphs (i)(3)(i) through (vi) of this section do not apply to buprenorphine and buprenorphine products listed under paragraph (h)(2)(iii) of this section.

(i) During the first 90 days of treatment, the take-home supply (beyond that of paragraph (i)(1) of this section) is limited to a single dose each week and the patient shall ingest all other doses under appropriate supervision as provided for under the regulations in this subpart.

(ii) In the second 90 days of treatment, the take-home supply (beyond that of paragraph (i)(1) of this section) are two doses per week.

(iii) In the third 90 days of treatment, the take-home supply (beyond that of paragraph (i)(1) of this section) are three doses per week.

(iv) In the remaining months of the first year, a patient may be given a maximum 6-day supply of take-home medication.

(v) After 1 year of continuous treatment, a patient may be given a maximum 2-week supply of take-home medication.

(vi) After 2 years of continuous treatment, a patient may be given a maximum one-month supply of take-home medication, but must make monthly visits.

(4) No medications shall be dispensed to patients in short-term detoxification treatment or interim maintenance treatment for unsupervised or take-home use.

(5) OTPs must maintain current procedures adequate to identify the theft or diversion of take-home medications, including labeling containers with the OTP's name, address, and telephone number. Programs also must ensure that take-home supplies are packaged in a manner that is designed to reduce the risk of accidental ingestion, including child-proof containers (see Poison Prevention Packaging Act, Public Law 91-601 (15 U.S.C. 1471*et seq.*)).

(j) *Interim maintenance treatment.*
(1) The program sponsor of a public or nonprofit private OTP may place an individual, who is eligible for admission to comprehensive maintenance treatment, in interim maintenance treatment if the individual cannot be placed in a public or nonprofit private comprehensive program within a reasonable geographic area and within 14 days of the individual's application for admission to comprehensive maintenance treatment. An initial and at least two other urine screens shall be taken from interim patients during the maximum of 120 days permitted for such treatment. A program shall establish and follow reasonable criteria for establishing priorities for transferring patients from interim maintenance to comprehensive maintenance treatment. These transfer criteria shall be in writing and shall include, at a minimum, a preference for pregnant women in admitting patients to interim maintenance and in transferring patientsfrom interim maintenance to comprehensive maintenance treatment. Interim maintenance shall be provided in a manner consistent with all applicable Federal and State laws, including sections 1923, 1927(a), and 1976 of the Public Health Service Act (21 U.S.C. 300x-23, 300x-27(a), and 300y-11).

(2) The program shall notify the State health officer when a patient begins interim maintenance treatment, when a patient leaves interim maintenance treatment, and before the date of mandatory transfer to a comprehensive program, and shall document such notifications.

(3) SAMHSA may revoke the interim maintenance authorization for programs that fail to comply with the provisions of this paragraph (j). Likewise, SAMHSA will consider revoking the interim maintenance authorization of a program if the State in which the program operates is not in compliance with the provisions of § 8.11(g).

(4) All requirements for comprehensive maintenance treatment apply to interim maintenance treatment with the following exceptions:

(i) The opioid agonist treatment medication is required to be administered daily under observation;

(ii) Unsupervised or "take-home" use is not allowed;

(iii) An initial treatment plan and periodic treatment plan evaluations are not required;

(iv) A primary counselor is not required to be assigned to the patient;

(v) Interim maintenance cannot be provided for longer than 120 days in any 12-month period; and

(vi) Rehabilitative, education, and other counseling services described in paragraphs (f)(4), (f)(5)(i), and (f)(5)(iii) of this section are not required to be provided to the patient.

[66 FR 4090, Jan. 17, 2001, as amended at 68 FR 27939, May 22, 2003; 77 FR 72761, Dec. 6, 2012; 80 FR 34838, June 18, 2015]

Appendix II

The ACEs Questionnaire (from: https://www.ncjfcj.org/sites/ default/files/Finding%20Your%20ACE%20Score.pdf)

Adverse Childhood Experience (ACE) Questionnaire Finding your ACE Score

While you were growing up, during your first 18 years of life:

1. Did a parent or other adult in the household **often** ...
   Swear at you, insult you, put you down, or humiliate you?

   or

   Act in a way that made you afraid that you might be physically hurt?

   Yes   No   If yes enter 1 _____

2. Did a parent or other adult in the household **often** ... Push, grab, slap, or throw something at you?

   or

   Ever hit you so hard that you had marks or were injured?

   Yes   No   If yes enter 1 _____

3. Did an adult or person at least 5 years older than you **ever**...
   Touch or fondle you or have you touch their body in a sexual way?

   or

   Try to or actually have oral, anal, or vaginal sex with you?

   Yes   No   If yes enter 1 _____

4. Did you **often** feel that ...
   No one in your family loved you or thought you were important or special?

   or

   Your family didn't look out for each other, feel close to each other, or support each other?

   Yes   No   If yes enter 1 _____

5. Did you **often** feel that ...
   You didn't have enough to eat, had to wear dirty clothes, and had no one to protect you?

   or

   Your parents were too drunk or high to take care of you or take you to the doctor if you needed it?

   Yes   No   If yes enter 1 _____

6. Were your parents **ever** separated or divorced?

   Yes   No   If yes enter 1 _____

7. Was your mother or stepmother:
Often pushed, grabbed, slapped, or had something thrown at her?

or

Sometimes or often kicked, bitten, hit with a fist, or hit with something hard?

or

Ever repeatedly hit over at least a few minutes or threatened with a gun or knife?

Yes   No   If yes enter 1 _____

8. Did you live with anyone who was a problem drinker or alcoholic or who used street drugs?

Yes   No   If yes enter 1 _____

9. Was a household member depressed or mentally ill or did a household member attempt suicide?

Yes   No   If yes enter 1 _____

10. Did a household member go to prison?
Yes   No   If yes enter 1 _____

Now add up your "Yes" answers: _____
This is your ACE Score

APPENDIX III

Glossary/Terminology

glucocorticoid – a class of steroid (cholesterol) based hormones that have wide-ranging effects on most every cell of the human body. *Cortisol* is the natural, endogenous glucocorticoid secreted in the human body. Prednisone is an example of a synthetic glucocorticoid. Whether natural or synthetic, glucocorticoids are absolutely essential for maintenance of the body's homeostatic mechanisms.

cortisol – the main natural, endogenous glucocorticoid secreted in the human body.

titration – the gradual process of adjusting a medication dosage upwards or downwards in order to arrive at an optimal dosage for that person.

SML (Serum Methadone Level) – a blood test that determines how much "free" methadone is circulating in the body. Unless it tests *stereo-selectively*, the information provided by this test can only be used to draw limited inferences as to how a given dosage affects a given individual.

stereo-selectivity – pertaining to the ability of a chemical test to individually determine quantitative differences (applied to the *SML*) between *chiral* molecules. A stereoselective SML can determine exactly how much of the active methadone molecule (l-methadone) is present in blood serum, and differentiate this from the inactive molecule (d-methadone.)

opioid agonist – any of a number of traditional opioids that elicits a full-effect from the *mu-opioid receptor*, some common examples being morphine, hydromorphone, heroin, oxycodone, methadone, fentanyl, etc.

opioid antagonist- any of a number of opioid-like (structurally) compounds that, like an *agonist*, binds to the opioid receptor, but opposes the effects of the activated receptor, and preferentially binds-to and blocks the receptor from eliciting any effect. Common examples include naloxone, naltrexone, and nalmefene. (WARNING: administration of an opioid antagonist to someone who is physically dependent on opioids will elicit a *violent, precipitated withdrawal syndrome.*)

partial opioid agonist/antagonist – as the term implies, these compounds exhibit pharmacological properties on a continuum somewhere between those of a full agonist and those of a full antagonist. Buprenorphine is the most familiar example of such a compound. (WARNING: administration of buprenorphine to someone who is still physically dependent may elicit a *precipitated withdrawal syndrome.* This is still one of the limitations of this compound that prevents its' more widespread use.)

naloxone, naltrexone, nalmefene – three of the most common *opioid antagonists* on the market. Naloxone has a very short duration of action, and must be given repeatedly (only by injection, infusion, or nasal spray) in order to fully reverse an overdose. Naltrexone can be taken orally and lasts for circa 36 hours, nalmefene can be injected and also has a long duration of action (virtually guaranteeing that overdose will be reversed, but not without potential adverse reactions.)

precipitated withdrawal syndrome – similar to the more standard, slow withdrawal, as its name implies, only in *quality* of symptoms, precipitated withdrawal is characterized by severe and far more intense withdrawal symptoms produced when there is a **precipitous** drop of either, 1) opioid present at the receptor, or 2) blood serum levels of opioid in the body.

This syndrome can (and has been) so severe so as to sometimes require emergency medical support and treatment.

ligand-receptor complex – the actual drug bound directly to its receptor, usually causing "downstream" effects from the thusly activated receptor.

half-life (pharmacology) – the amount of time required for the body to remove half of the original dosage from the body. Can be viewed as a rough proxy for the relative duration of the drug's persistence in the body/duration of therapeutic effect.

chirality – a concept in organic chemistry that arises from the unique way that carbon can bond with other atoms. Derived from the Greek word for "hand," it describes the stereo-like "handedness" of many different organic compounds. As it relates to methadone, this medication exists as a 50:50 mixture of l-methadone (the actual, working opioid) and d-methadone (opioid inactive, mirror-image of l-methadone.) Think of a right hand and a left hand: They are at once the same (identical construction of parts) and yet still different (mirror-images of each other that cannot be superimposed upon one another.)

neurotypical – A neurotypical person is an individual who thinks, perceives, and behaves in ways that are considered to be "normal" by the general population.

MAT – Medication Assisted Treatment
MMT – Methadone Maintenance Treatment
AATOD – American Association for the Treatment of Opioid Disorders
ASAM – American Society for Addiction Medicine
ACE's – Adverse Childhood Experiences
CDC – Centers for Disease Control
PAWS – Post Acute Withdrawal Syndrome

mu, delta, and kappa opioid receptors – In the human brain, there are 3 main types of opioid receptor. Most important for this discussion, by far, is the mu-opioid receptor, for it is mostly responsible for the psychoactive, especially euphoric and analgesic, effects of most opioid agonists. Delta and kappa receptors also play important roles themselves as part of the entire endogenous opioid system; any further discussion is beyond the scope of this text.

Appendix IV

CDC OPIOID GUIDELINES 2016

The following is a small excerpt from the 2016 guidelines issued by the CDC regarding opioid analgesic prescription, as the full document is almost a book in itself, and the very most pertinent problems with the guidelines are fully contained within this excerpt;

- Start with the lowest effective dose and carefully evaluate risks and benefits before increasing to 50 morphine milligram equivalents (MME)/day (MME = MED = morphine equianalgesic dose)
- Increase frequency of follow-up (every 3 months max) or consider offering naloxone
- *Avoid increasing to >90 MME/day*
- If still no relief of pain, *consider tapering to a lower dose or discontinue* [100]

An explanation of the italicized clauses is needed in order to faithfully depict the agony (and deaths by suicide) that have resulted from the DEA concurrently placing a proverbial boot on the neck of every physician in the U.S., apparently to make sure that the "suggestions" will be followed *no matter the outcome to the patient.* [146]

MME stands for Morphine Milligram Equivalents, and without getting too involved in the granular details, MME/day is written as an absolute maximum ("avoid increasing to >90 MME/day") per patient, per day. For the record, 90 mg. of morphine (or its' equivalent) per day (orally taken) is a small dose for a chronic pain patient and, depending upon the injury, can even be considered a relatively small dose limit for some patients with acute pain (i.e., patients with no established tolerance to opioids).

From one day to the next, patients who had been taking >90 MME/day (which happened to most often be chronic pain patients treated for years at a higher, but steady and unchanging dose) were unceremoniously "shown the door" by their respective physicians. Just as an example, most chronic pain patients had been well-maintained on *150-1,000 MME/day...*

From the day the 2016 CDC Guidelines were released, an ever-increasing proportion of physicians began to interpret this "suggested" upper limit on daily opioid dose as an absolute imperative. This is empirically derived from the sequelae that ensued shortly after the guidelines were released.

With an alarming, steady increase in physicians' attempts to legally protect their licenses to practice medicine came the phenomena of either, 1) Drastic and rapid dose-reduction of opioid analgesics that had been prescribed (in many cases) for years to chronic pain patients down to the 90 MME suggested upper limit for daily dosage, *if the patient was lucky*, or, 2) An immediate cessation of any further opioid prescription. Period. No weaning, gradual reduction, etc., just leaving the opioid dependent patients to fend for themselves.

Important to bear-in-mind is that the current hysteria that has enveloped all pain patients, in spite of the CDC's insistence that the guidelines were *only* "suggestions" for chronic non-malignant pain, is now *de facto* adversely affecting *all people in the U.S.* needing to be treated for moderate-to-severe pain, be it acute, chronic, and even cancer pain and palliative care. This is a classic example of "throwing out the baby with the bath water," and the few clauses listed here (especially those that have been italicized) are the *direct cause* of an unimaginable amount of needless human suffering happening right now across the country. [146]

If physicians lose their DEA privileges, it is essentially identical (in end-effect) to losing their license to practice medicine, so it is not all that surprising that most American physicians have taken these guidelines as being, again, *de facto* directives. The victims of all of this heavy-handedness are "only" pain patients of all stripes (acute, chronic, post-surgical, cancer, terminal illness, etc.), not the physicians, nor the DEA, nor the legislators, who have done more than their part in creating this problem.

Of course, legislators tend to be protected from such medical extremes simply by virtue of their *position and power* relative to the average citizen. It's no secret that legislators get the best healthcare that taxpayer dollars can provide. So why is it that they are exempt (literally) from the agony that other, less powerful citizens can no longer avoid? [146]

What to do about such an adverse situation, particularly when there is such an imbalance of power between the two groups who are now locked in a *de facto* adversarial stance toward one another? There are no clear answers, but there is an intuitive sense that only when pain patients, as a group, *sponsor a Washington, D.C. lobbyist*, will their cries finally be heard and, most crucially, be answered appropriately.

APPENDIX V

Author interview with Dr. Robert Sapolsky, Ph.D.
(Stanford University)

Dr. Sapolsky, thank you very much for getting back to me. The questions I have for you relate to the intersection between chemical addiction, specifically opioid addiction, and the brain. I am noting the clear and absolute distinctions between opioid addiction (rare) and opioid dependence (much more common, and a normal part of everyday medical practice).

1-Do you subscribe to the hypothesis that there is an organic, physiological predisposition for the development of opioid addiction?

Yes, but this isn't too helpful of an answer from me, in that I believe that there is an organic physiological predisposition for most, if not all of our traits and vulnerabilities.

2-Given that opioid addiction (vs dependence) most resembles chronic diseases like diabetes, Crohn's, and hypertension do you believe that there is a permanent brain alteration (e.g. in connectivity between PFC and limbic system) by opioids, ultimately rendering "abstinence-based" treatments ineffectual in the long term?

3-Since the early 2000's, there have been a number of genetic association studies of various polymorphisms of certain potentially important genes such as the OPRM1 mu-opioid receptor SNP rs1799971 (A118G), or the ABCB1-blood-brain barrier efflux pump "gene", for example. What do you make of these studies, and what (if anything) do they tell us about the heritability of opioid addiction?

The previous to [*sic*] questions are ones that are out of my league, definitely.

4-When considering the CDC's original Adverse Childhood Experience's study, what relative role do ACE's have, particularly as the number of adverse events increase, on the development of opioid addiction in vulnerable individuals?

I suspect there are a bunch of paths from lots of ACEs to adult addiction – for example, the fact that a lot of ACEs effects frontal cortical development in a way that make people very steep temporal discounters – why wait for a good reward tomorrow when you can have an unhealthy one now? For my money, I think the biggest effects of ACEs is via stress effects on development of the dopamine system – predisposing individuals towards depression and anxiety (and with the resulting increased odds of falling into self-medicating), and making for a system that is, in general, less responsive to typical rewards.

5-Is the nature of the vulnerability-factor with addicts so great that said individuals, if exposed to the right environment, will become addicts *irrespective of their psychological histories*?

It's probably something akin to the trauma literature, where there are people whose biological vulnerability is so high that they are flattened by the smallest of challenges, and people whose bilogical resilience is so great that they come out of the Holocaust relatively psychologically intact.

6-With reference to the aforementioned ACE's, what mediating role do you feel glucocorticoids (and also CRH) have with respect to the resultant increased morbidity and mortality, irrespective of whether or not the affected individual goes on to opioid addiction or not?

A tremendous role, particularly in terms of the effects of glucocorticoids (and CRH) on the developing brain.

7-How do you feel about treating opioid addiction as a chronic, relapsing, *physically* based disease, with indefinite substitution therapy vs abstinence based approaches?

This one's out of my expertise, definitely.
These responses are definitely on the record.

Hope this is helpful,
Robert Sapolsky

REFERENCES

FOR: "The Enlightened Guide To Methadone Maintenance Treatment: A Handbook for Navigating Opiate Addiction through Methadone Maintenance Treatment for Providers, Patients and their Families", Borzsony, Kay John

1) Long-Acting Injectable Naltrexone for the Management of Patients with Opioid Dependence 2011, https://www.ncbi.nlm.nih.gov/pmc/articles/PMC3411517/

2) Use of Naltrexone to Treat Opioid Addiction in a Country in Which Methadone and Buprenorphine Are Not Available2010, https://www.ncbi.nlm.nih.gov/pmc/articles/PMC3160743/

3) p.6, National Practice Guideline for the Use of Medications in the Treatment of Addiction Involving Opioid Use, ASAM 2015, https://www.asam.org/docs/default-source/practice-support/guidelines-and-consensus-docs/asam-national-practice-guideline-supplement.pdf

4) Is levorphanol a better option than methadone?, https://academic.oup.com/painmedicine/article/16/9/1673/1875439

5) Fischer 344 and Lewis Rat Strains as a Model of Genetic Vulnerability to Drug Addiction, https://www.ncbi.nlm.nih.gov/pmc/articles/PMC4746315/

6) Adverse Childhood Experiences: Risk Factors for Substance Misuse and Mental Health (video), https://www.samhsa.gov/capt/tools-learning-resources/aces-risk-factors-substance-misuse

7) The adverse childhood experiences questionnaire: Two decades of research on childhood trauma as a primary cause of adult mental illness, addiction, and medical diseases, https://www.tandfonline.com/doi/full/10.1080/2331205X.2019.1581447

8) Maintenance Medication for Opiate Addiction: The Foundation of Recovery, https://www.ncbi.nlm.nih.gov/pmc/articles/PMC3411273/

9) The History of the Original ACEs Study, https://www.osymigrant. org/ACES/Chapter%20Two%20The%20History%20of%20the%20 Original%20ACEs%20Study.pdf

10) The Role of Adverse Childhood Experiences in Substance Misuse and Related Behavioral Health Problems, https://www.samhsa.gov/capt/ sites/default/files/resources/aces-behavioral-health-problems.pdf

11) Author interview with Dr. Robert Sapolsky (Stanford), personal communications, Tuesday, January 15, 2019

12) "60% fewer insurers cover opioid addiction drugs now than in 2007 – but almost all cover the painkillers fueling the overdose epidemic, study finds the number of people dying of opioid overdoses has surged since the 1990s", https://www.dailymail.co.uk/health/article-6695799/60-fewer-insurers-cover-opioid-addiction-drugs-2007-study-finds.html

13) FDA Says Benzodiazepine Use Not a Bar to Treatment with Methadone or Buprenorphine for opioid, http://atforum.com/2017/10/fda-says-benzodiazepine-use-not-a-bar-to-treatment-with-methadone-or-buprenorphine-for-opioid-addiction/

14) FDA Drug Safety Communications, 9/20/2017, https://www.fda.gov/ downloads/Drugs/DrugSafety/UCM576377.pdf

15) AATOD Guidelines for Addressing Benzodiazepine Use in Opioid Treatment Programs (OTPs), http://www.aatod.org/guidelines-for-addressing-benzodiazepine-use-in-opioid-treatment-programs-otps/

16) FDA: Use of Buprenorphine and Methadone With Benzodiazepines Is OK-Benefits of opioid addiction treatment outweigh risks of adverse effects,https://www.managedcaremag.com/news/fda-use-buprenorphine-and-methadone-benzodiazepines-ok

17) "Methadonia" (film), https://behavenet.com/methadonia

18) "Doctors Who Hate Drug Users Are Fueling the Opioid Crisis: SPOS—or subhuman piece of shit—is old hospital slang for drug users. That attitude is still all over America's response to a drug epidemic." https://www.vice.com/en_us/article/43nzyq/doctors-who-hate-drug-users-are-fueling-the-opioid-crisis

19) "What's Missing from the National Discussion About the Opioid Epidemic" https://www.newyorker.com/tech/annals-of-technology/whats-missing-national-discussion-opioid-epidemic

20) "Creating the American Junkie: Addiction Research in the Classic Era of Narcotic Control", Acker, Caroline Jean, 2006, Johns Hopkins University Press, Baltimore

21) Chronic Stress, Drug Use, and Vulnerability to Addiction (2008), https://www.ncbi.nlm.nih.gov/pmc/articles/PMC2732004/

22) Inter-individual variability of the clinical pharmacokinetics of methadone: implications for the treatment of opioid dependence, Eap et.al., Clinical Pharmacokinetics. 2002;41(14):1153-93., PMID: 12405865, https://www.ncbi.nlm.nih.gov/pubmed/12405865

23) "Chasing The Scream", Hari, Johann, 2016, Bloomsbury Publishing, USA

24) Commonly Prescribed Meds for Treating Addiction Also Reduce Crime and Suicide, https://www.medscape.com/viewarticle/907874

25) Treatment and Prevention of Opioid Use Disorder: Challenges and Opportunities, https://www.ncbi.nlm.nih.gov/pmc/articles/PMC5880741/

26) International Stakeholder Community of Pain Experts and Leaders Call for an Urgent Action on Forced Opioid Tapering, https://academic.oup.com/painmedicine/advance-article/doi/10.1093/pm/pny228/5218985

27) *In The Realm of Hungry Ghosts: Close Encounters with Addiction*, Mate, Gabor, 2008, North Atlantic Books, Berkeley, CA

28) "When 'Enough' is not Enough", Maxwell, Shindermann, Leavitt, Eap https://wmich.edu/sites/default/files/attachments/u372/2015/When%20Enough%20Is%20Not%20Enough.pdf

29) Part B: 20 Questions and Answers Regarding Methadone Maintenance Treatment Research, NIDA International Program, Methadone Research Web Guide, https://www.drugabuse.gov/sites/default/files/pdf/partb.pdf

30) Methadone Dose-capping Still Continues in Practice, If Not in Policy2015 http://atforum.com/2015/06/methadone-dose-capping-still-continues-in-practice-if-not-in-policy/

31) "Methadone dosing and safety in the Tx of addiction", AT Forum, http://atforum.com/documents/DosingandSafetyWP.pdf

32) Treating Drug Problems: Volume 1: A Study of the Evolution, Effectiveness, and Financing of Public and Private Drug Treatment Systems- The Effectiveness of Treatment, https://www.ncbi.nlm.nih.gov/books/NBK235506/

33) High dose versus moderate dose methadone maintenance: is there a better outcome? https://www.ncbi.nlm.nih.gov/pubmed/20155609

34) Ethnic and genetic factors in methadone pharmacokinetics: A population pharmacokinetic study, https://www.ncbi.nlm.nih.gov/pmc/articles/PMC4254688/

35) ASAM Statement on Pharmacological Therapies for Opioid Use Disorders(2013),https://www.asam.org/advocacy/find-a-policy-statement/view-policy-statement/public-policy-statements/2013/04/25/pharmacological-therapies-for-opioid-use-disorders

36) AATOD Statement-Using Medication Assisted Treatment to Treat Opioid Use Disorder: Learning from Past Experience to Guide Policy, http://www.aatod.org/wp-content/uploads/2019/02/2019-Policy-Paper.pdf

37) Incarceration and opioid withdrawal: The experiences of methadone patients and out-of-treatment heroin users, http://www.ncbi.nlm.nih.gov/pmc/articles/PMC2838492/

38) Cellular neuroadaptations to chronic opioids: tolerance, withdrawal and addiction, https://bpspubs.onlinelibrary.wiley.com/doi/full/10.1038/bjp.2008.100

39) ASAM Statement on Pharmacological Therapies for Opioid Use Disorders(2013),https://www.asam.org/advocacy/find-a-policy-statement/view-policy-statement/public-policy-statements/2013/04/25/pharmacological-therapies-for-opioid-use-disorders

40) Dole, V.P.; Nyswander, M.E. and Kreek, M.J. Narcotic blockade. Archives of Internal Medicine 1966 118: 304-309., https://www.ncbi.nlm.nih.gov/pubmed/4162686

41) Implications of Methadone Maintenance for Theories of Narcotic Addiction, by Vincent P. Dole M.D., Dole, V. JAMA 1988 Vol. 260:

3025-3029., http://www.methadone.org/downloads/documents/1988_
dole_jama_implications_of_mm_theories_of_addiction.pdf

42) Heroin Addiction – A Metabolic Disease, *Vincent P. Dole, MD and
Marie E. Nyswander, MD, New York Arch Intern Med–Vol 120,
July 1967,* http://www.doraweiner.com/dole_nyswander_1967.pdf

43) Opioid Overdose: Understanding the Epidemic, https://www.cdc.gov/
drugoverdose/epidemic/index.html

44) Federal Regulation of Methadone Treatment, https://www.ncbi.nlm.
nih.gov/books/NBK232105/

45) Ex-Addicts Find Methadone More Elusive Than Heroin, *New York
Times*, Feb.2, 1997, https://www.nytimes.com/1997/02/02/us/ex-
addicts-find-methadone-more-elusive-than-heroin.html

46) Methadone Maintenance 4 Decades Later2008, https://jamanetwork.
com/journals/jama/fullarticle/182898

47) PROPOSAL FOR THE INCLUSION OF METHADONE IN THE
WHO MODEL LIST OF ESSENTIAL MEDICINES, https://www.
who.int/substance_abuse/activities/methadone_essential_medicines.
pdf

48) The Real Gateway Drug Isn't Marijuana, http://www.thea
tlantic.com/health/archive/2015/04/the-real-gateway-drug-
isnt-marijuana/391266/

49) Commentary: Countering the Myths About Methadone (Dr. Salsitz),
https://drugfree.org/learn/drug-and-alcohol-news/commentary-
countering-the-myths-about-methadone/

50) Piaget's theory of cognitive development (entry), www.Wikipedia.org

51) U.S. Jails Are Killing People Going Through Opioid Withdrawals,
https://www.huffingtonpost.com/the-influence/us-jails-are-killing-
people-opioid-withdrawals_b_9563940.html

52) Go to Jail. Die From Drug Withdrawal. Welcome to the Criminal
Justice System, https://www.motherjones.com/politics/2017/02/
opioid-withdrawal-jail-deaths/

53) Moderate- vs High-Dose Methadone in the Treatment of Opioid
Dependence-ARandomizedTrial1999,https://www.ncbi.nlm.nih.gov/
pubmed/20155609, https://jamanetwork.com/journals/jama/fullarticle/189103

54) AT Forum: Dosage Survey '98: Changes for the Better, www.atforum.com

55) Variations in Methadone Treatment practices, 1992, JAMA, www. JAMA.com/archives

56) High-Dose Methadone Improves Treatment Outcomes, https:// archives.drugabuse.gov/news-events/nida-notes/1999/12/high-dose-methadone-improves-treatment-outcomes

57) TENNESSEE DEPT. OF MENTAL HEALTH, MINIMUM PROGRAM REQUIREMENTS FOR NON-RESIDENTIAL OPIOID TREATMENT PROGRAM FACILITIES, https://publications. tnsosfiles.com/rules/0940/0940-05/0940-05-42.20121219.pdf

58) Trump's budget proposal does nothing for the opioid epidemic2019, https://www.vox.com/policy-and-politics/2019/3/11/18260152/ trump-budget-opioid-epidemic-2019

59) Trouble Ahead: Shifts in Funding Limit Access to Methadone, Threaten Treatment Expansion, February 21, 2019, http://atforum.com/2019/02/ funding-limit-access-methadone-threaten-treatment-expansion/

60) ASAM Public Policy Statement on Office-based Opioid Agonist Treatment (OBOT), https://www.asam.org/docs/default-source/public-policy-statements/1obot-treatment-7-04.pdf?sfvrsn=0

61) *The Protectors: Harry J. Anslinger and the Federal Bureau of Narcotics, 1930-62*, Newark, DE: University of Delaware Press, McWilliams, John C.

62) How Racial Bias Has Shaped the Opioid Epidemic, https://www. usnews.com/news/healthiest-communities/articles/2019-02-11/ racism-helped-shape-the-opioid-epidemic-study-suggests

63) OpioidsandHepatitisC:HowOxyContinFedaNewEpidemic(unintended consequencesofreformulation),https://ldi.upenn.edu/healthpolicysense/ opioids-and-hepatitis-c-how-oxycontin-fed-new-epidemic

64) Drugs, Brains, and Behavior: The Science of Addiction, https://www. drugabuse.gov/publications/drugs-brains-behavior-science-addiction/ drugs-brain

65) The New Jim Crow, Alexander, Michelle

66) Data and Maps: Excessive Drinking, https://www.cdc.gov/alcohol/ data-stats.htm

67) ASAM Joint Public Correctional Policy Statement on the Treatment of Opioid Use Disorders for Justice Involved Individuals, https://www.asam.org/advocacy/find-a-policy-statement/view-policy-statement/public-policy-statements/2018/03/20/joint-public-correctional-policy-statement-on-the-treatment-of-opioid-use-disorders-for-justice-involved-individuals

68) Forced Jailhouse Withdrawal, http://www.ncbi.nlm.nih.gov/pmc/articles/PMC2838492/

69) When Going to Jail Means Giving Up The Meds That Saved Your Life, https://www.themarshallproject.org/2019/01/29/when-going-to-jail-means-giving-up-the-meds-that-saved-your-life

70) Dying by detox: Heroin-related jail deaths raise alarm with advocates, https://www.cbsnews.com/news/heroin-withdrawal-jail-deaths-treatment-advocates/]

71) Death by detox, http://america.aljazeera.com/opinions/2015/10/death-by-detox.html

72) Forced withdrawal from methadone maintenance therapy in criminal justice settings: A critical treatment barrier in the United States, https://www.ncbi.nlm.nih.gov/pmc/articles/PMC3695471/

73) Inmate dies 'excruciating' death from drug withdrawal in Macomb County Jail, https://www.mlive.com/news/detroit/2015/09/inmate_dies_excruciating_death.html

74) FBI investigating inmate's death from drug withdrawal in Macomb County Jail, https://www.mlive.com/news/detroit/2015/09/fbi_investigating_jail_death_o.html

75) 18 people have died in the Macomb County Jail since 2012. This is one woman's story., https://www.michiganradio.org/post/18-people-have-died-macomb-county-jail-2012-one-womans-story

76) Macomb County Jail inmate suicide sparks lawsuit, https://www.detroitnews.com/story/news/local/macomb-county/2019/07/29/macomb-county-jail-inmate-suicide-sparks-lawsuit/1844814001/

77) Federal officials decline to file charges in Macomb inmate's death, https://www.detroitnews.com/story/news/local/macomb-county/2016/09/19/federal-charges-denied-macomb-jail-death/90699630/

78) Notable Individuals who Succumb to Relapse http://styleblazer.com/159698/they-slipped-after-treatment-14-late-life-celebs-who-experienced-a-relapse/

79) SINCE SANDRA: Here are the 815 people (and counting) who have lost their lives in jail in the year after Sandra Bland died., http://data.huffingtonpost.com/2016/jail-deaths

80) The potential risks and high cost of using opioid blocking drugs during heavy sedation or anesthesia to bring on withdrawal outweigh the benefits, https://www.cochrane.org/CD002022/ADDICTN_the-potential-risks-and-high-cost-of-using-opioid-blocking-drugs-during-heavy-sedation-or-anaesthesia-to-bring-on-withdrawal-outweigh-the-benefits

81) Evidence-Based Addiction Treatment vs. Ultra-Rapid Detox: The problem with ultra-rapid detox – Beware, https://www.naabt.org/urod.cfm

82) Public Policy Statement on Rapid and Ultra Rapid Opioid Detoxification, https://www.asam.org/advocacy/find-a-policy-statement/view-policy-statement/public-policy-statements/2011/12/15/rapid-and-ultra-rapid-opioid-detoxification

83) Morbidity and Mortality Weekly Report: Deaths and Severe Adverse Events Associated with Anesthesia-Assisted Rapid Opioid Detoxification—New York City, 2012, https://www.cdc.gov/mmwr/preview/mmwrhtml/mm6238a1.htm

84) Complications of Ultra-rapid Opioid Detoxification with Subcutaneous Naltrexone Pellets, https://onlinelibrary.wiley.com/doi/abs/10.1197/aemj.9.1.63

85) Cellular basis of memory for addiction2013, https://www.ncbi.nlm.nih.gov/pmc/articles/PMC3898681/

86) Genetics of Opioid Dependence: A Review of the Genetic Contribution to Opioid Dependence2014, https://www.ncbi.nlm.nih.gov/pmc/articles/PMC4155832/

87) Genetic and Familial Environmental Influences on the Risk for Drug Abuse: A National Swedish Adoption Study2012 https://www.ncbi.nlm.nih.gov/pmc/articles/PMC3556483/

88) Affective neuroscience of pleasure: reward in humans and animals 2010, https://www.ncbi.nlm.nih.gov/pmc/articles/PMC3004012/

89) Cellular neuroadaptations to chronic opioids: tolerance, withdrawal and addiction, https://bpspubs.onlinelibrary.wiley.com/doi/full/10.1038/bjp.2008.100

90) Introducing Precision Addiction Management of Reward Deficiency Syndrome, the Construct That Underpins All Addictive Behaviors, https://www.ncbi.nlm.nih.gov/pmc/articles/PMC6277779/

91) Endogenous Opioid System Dysregulation in Depression: Implications for New Therapeutic Approaches, https://www.ncbi.nlm.nih.gov/pmc/articles/PMC6310672/

92) Response of the μ-opioid system to social rejection and acceptance, https://www.ncbi.nlm.nih.gov/pmc/articles/PMC3814222/

93) It still hurts: altered opioid activity in the brain during social rejection and acceptance in major depressive disorder, https://www.ncbi.nlm.nih.gov/pmc/articles/PMC4469367/

94) Early-life adversity facilitates acquisition of cocaine self-administration and induces persistent anhedonia, https://www.ncbi.nlm.nih.gov/pmc/articles/PMC5991313/

95) Long-Term Associations of Justice Sensitivity, Rejection Sensitivity, and Depressive Symptoms in Children and Adolescents, https://www.ncbi.nlm.nih.gov/pmc/articles/PMC5601073/

96) Distinctive Profiles of Gene Expression in the Human Nucleus Accumbens Associated with Cocaine and Heroin Abuse, https://www.ncbi.nlm.nih.gov/pmc/articles/PMC2239258/

97) Ventral striatal regulation of CREM mediates impulsive action and drug addiction vulnerability, https://www.ncbi.nlm.nih.gov/pmc/articles/PMC5656565/

98) Dopamine-dependent responses to morphine depend on glucocorticoid receptors, https://www.ncbi.nlm.nih.gov/pmc/articles/PMC22744/

99) Trauma-Informed Approaches Need to be Part of a Comprehensive Strategy for Addressing the Opioid Epidemic, https://publichealth.gwu.edu/sites/default/files/downloads/Redstone-Center/CTIPP_OPB_final.pdf

100) Opioids & Early Adversity: Connecting Childhood Trauma and Addiction, http://www.ncsl.org/portals/1/documents/health/Opioid Webinar_32211.pdf

101) ACES & OPIATES: Connecting the Impact of Adverse Childhood Experiences on Addiction, http://www.bbahc.org/vertical/sites/% 7BD98FECDC-9EAF-4437-8F06-33DC6FAF263C%7D/uploads/ Substance_Abuse_Issues_-_What_You_Need_to_Know.pdf

102) Adverse childhood experience effects on opioid use initiation, injection drug use, and overdose among persons with opioid use disorder, https://europepmc.org/articles/pmc5599365

103) Early Adverse Experiences and the Developing Brain, *Neuropsychopharmacology.* 2016 Jan; 41(1): 177–196., https://europepmc.org/ articles/PMC4677140/

104) The enduring effects of abuse and related adverse experiences in childhood- A convergence of evidence from neurobiology and epidemiology, *European Archives of Psychiatry and Clinical Neuroscience.* 2006 Apr; 256(3): 174–186., https://europepmc.org/ articles/PMC3232061/

105) The Origins of Addiction: Evidence from the Adverse Childhood Experiences Study, Vincent J. Felitti, M.D., Department of Preventive Medicine, Kaiser Permanente Medical Care Program, San Diego, CA, https://www.nijc.org/pdfs/Subject%20Matter%20Articles/Drugs%20 and%20Alc/ACE%20Study%20-%20OriginsofAddiction.pdf

106) Behave, Robert M. Sapolsky, 2017, Penguin Press, ISBN 9781594205071

107) The 2016 CDC Opioid Prescribing Guidelines, https://www. cdc.gov/mmwr/volumes/65/rr/rr6501e1.htm?CDC_AA_refVal= https%3A%2F%2Fwww.cdc.gov%2Fmmwr%2Fvolumes%2F65%2 Frr%2Frr6501e1er.htm

108) Request for Civil Rights Investigation into Macomb County Jail and "Pay or Stay" Sentencing, https://www.aclumich.org/sites/default/ files/ACLULettertoGuptaandDeClercqWithExhibit.pdf

109) FBIdocumentsrevealnewdetailsaboutinmate'sdeathatMacombCounty Jail, https://www.clickondetroit.com/news/2017/10/24/fbi-documents-reveal-new-details-about-inmates-death-at-macomb-county-jail/

110) David Stojcevski's horrifying death in jail, explained, https://www. vox.com/2015/9/26/9399391/macomb-county-jail-david-stojcevski

111) Physical Dependence and Addiction: An Important Distinction, http:// www.naabt.org/addiction_physical-dependence.cfm/

112) The Words We Choose Matter, http://www.naabt.org/language/

113) Letter to the CDC from HP3 March 6, 2019, https://docs.google. com/document/d/1RzQDSppUKhjiAsEmhW2WbTXlP5V8vJ4M_ vBPQLKhK_8/edit [HP3=Health Professionals for Patients in Pain; signed by 300 noted physicians]

114) The Feds Are About to Stick It to Pain Patients in a Big Way-Doctors are already getting spooked out of prescribing painkillers, and new rules could make life in some of America's struggling communities even worse, https://www.vice.com/en_us/article/8qb4dg/the-feds-are-about-to-stick-it-to-pain-patients-in-a-big-way

115) Pain Patients to Congress: CDC's Opioid Guideline Is Hurting Us—Has stoked "climate of fear" leading to inadequate treatment of chronic pain, https://www.medpagetoday.com/primarycare/opioids/77996

116) Big Pharma Targeted at Senate Hearing on Opioid Crisis—Sen. Durbin questions need to make 14 billion opioid doses per year, https:// www.medpagetoday.com/psychiatry/addictions/78302?xid=nl_mpt_ DHE_2019-03-01&eun=g1190747d0r&utm_source=Sailthru&utm_ medium=email&utm_campaign=NEW%20Daily%20Headlines%20 Email_TestB%202019-03-01&utm_term=Serif%20Daily%20 Headlines%20Email%20TestB

117) Doctors Who Hate Drug Users Are Fueling the Opioid Crisis: SPOS—or subhuman piece of shit—is old hospital slang for drug users. That attitude is still all over America's response to a drug epidemic, https://www.vice.com/en_us/article/43nzyq/doctors-who-hate-drug-users-are-fueling-the-opioid-crisis

118) How the Reformulation of OxyContin Ignited the Heroin Epidemic, https://www.cato.org/publications/research-briefs-economic-policy/how-reformulation-oxycontin-ignited-heroin-epidemic

119) Outdated drug policies leave millions of Africans in agony-The war on drugs has hurt patients who need painkillers, https://

www.economist.com/middle-east-and-africa/2019/02/02/
outdated-drug-policies-leave-millions-of-africans-in-agony

120) Federal Regulation of Methadone Treatment, Treatment Standards and Optimal Treatment, https://www.ncbi.nlm.nih.gov/books/NBK232109/

121) "Dear PROP/CDC, Here's What Happens When You Over-Restrict Pills: More Deaths. Nice Going.", https://www.acsh.org/news/2018/12/12/dear-propcdc-heres-what-happens-when-you-over-restrict-pills-more-deaths-nice-going-13663

122) "Who Is Telling The Truth About Prescription Opioid Deaths? DEA? CDC? Neither?", https://www.acsh.org/news/2018/11/05/who-telling-truth-about-prescription-opioid-deaths-dea-cdc-neither-13569

123) 'Study Links Rising Heroin Deaths to 2010 OxyContin Reformulation.' DUH!, https://www.acsh.org/news/2018/04/09/study-links-rising-heroin-deaths-2010-oxycontin-reformulation-duh-12812

124) Survey Shows Doctors Shunning Pain Patients, https://www.painnewsnetwork.org/stories/2017/3/14/survey-shows-doctors-shunning-chronic-pain-patients

125) The Relationship Between Chronic Pain and Suicide-Related Outcomes (V.A.), https://www.hsrd.research.va.gov/for_researchers/cyber_seminars/archives/2276-notes.pdf

126) Intracranial Self-Stimulation to Evaluate Abuse Potential of Drugs, https://www.ncbi.nlm.nih.gov/pmc/articles/PMC4081730/

127) Forced withdrawal from methadone maintenance therapy in criminal justice settings: A critical treatment barrier in the United States, https://www.ncbi.nlm.nih.gov/pmc/articles/PMC3695471/

128) Jail Ordered to Give Inmate Methadone for Opioid Addiction in Far-Reaching Ruling, https://www.nytimes.com/2018/11/28/us/inmate-methadone-opioid-addiction-ruling.html

129) Meta-analysis of drug-related deaths soon after release from prison, https://www.ncbi.nlm.nih.gov/pmc/articles/PMC2955973/

130) Methadone continuation versus forced withdrawal on incarceration in a combined U.S. prison and jail: a randomized, open-label trial, https://www.ncbi.nlm.nih.gov/pmc/articles/PMC4522212/

131) Opioid substitution therapy as a strategy to reduce deaths in prison: retrospective cohort study, https://bmjopen.bmj.com/content/4/4/e004666

132) A prison system offered all inmates addiction treatment. Overdose deaths dropped sharply, https://www.statnews.com/2018/02/14/medication-assisted-treatment-inmates/

133) Methadone maintenance in prison results in treatment retention, lower drug usage following release, https://www.drugabuse.gov/news-events/news-releases/2015/05/methadone-maintenance-in-prison-results-in-treatment-retention-lower-drug-usage-following-release

134) Moving Ahead on Methadone in Corrections, http://atforum.com/2018/02/moving-ahead-on-methadone-in-corrections/

135) N.I.H. Consensus Statement 1997: Effective Medical Treatment of Opiate Addiction, https://consensus.nih.gov/1997/1998TreatOpiateAddiction108PDF.pdf

136) Krokodil: The drug that eats junkies, https://www.independent.co.uk/news/world/europe/krokodil-the-drug-that-eats-junkies-2300787.html

137) Krokodil: how 'flesh-eating zombie drug' is causing a global crisis, http://theconversation.com/krokodil-how-flesh-eating-zombie-drug-is-causing-a-global-crisis-106371

138) Author's personal experiences (2000-2020)

139) Treatment and Prevention of Opioid Use Disorder: Challenges and Opportunities, https://www.ncbi.nlm.nih.gov/pmc/articles/PMC5880741/

140) Methadone Maintenance Facts, https://baartprograms.com/methadone-maintenance-facts/

141) Primary care physicians' perspectives on the prescription opioid epidemic, https://www.ncbi.nlm.nih.gov/pmc/articles/PMC4939126/

142) 2014 Survey Finds Physicians May View Opioid-Addicted Patients Negatively, https://www.practicalpainmanagement.com/treatments/addiction-medicine/opioid-use-disorder/survey-finds-physicians-may-view-opioid-addicted

143) Internalized stigma as an independent risk factor for substance use problems among primary care patients: Rationale and preliminary support, https://www.ncbi.nlm.nih.gov/pmc/articles/PMC5648632/

144) Trump Promised Anti-Opioid 'Scare' Ads. Here Are the First 4. The ads are aimed at young adults and feature glimpses of graphic scenes., https://www.usnews.com/news/healthiest-communities/articles/2018-06-07/trump-administration-launches-scare-tv-ads-to-fight-opioid-abuse

145) Methadone, professional prescribing information, https://www.drugs.com/pro/methadone.html

146) Trends and Rapidity of Dose Tapering Among Patients Prescribed Long-term Opioid Therapy, 2008-2017, November 15, 2019, https://jamanetwork.com/journals/jamanetworkopen/fullarticle/2755492

147) "Methadone Maintenance Treatment in the U.S.", Wechsberg, Wendee and Kasten, Jennifer, Springer Publishing Company, New York, NY

Made in the USA
San Bernardino, CA
24 April 2020